Postnatal Depression and Maternal Mental Health

A handbook for front-line caregivers working with women with perinatal mental health difficulties

**Edited by
Sue Gellhorn**

Pavilion

Postnatal Depression and Maternal Mental Health

A handbook for frontline caregivers working with women with perinatal mental health difficulties

Published by:
Pavilion Publishing and Media Ltd
Rayford House
School Road
Hove
East Sussex
BN3 5HX
Tel: 01273 434 943
Fax: 01273 227 308
Email: info@pavpub.com

Published 2016

A catalogue record for this book is available from the British Library.

ISBN: 978-1-910366-29-5

Pavilion is the leading training and development provider and publisher in the health, social care and allied fields, providing a range of innovative training solutions underpinned by sound research and professional values. We aim to put our customers first, through excellent customer service and value.

Author: Sue Gellhorn
Production editor: Ruth Chalmers, Pavilion Publishing and Media Ltd.
Cover design: Emma Dawe, Pavilion Publishing and Media Ltd.
Page layout and typesetting: Emma Dawe, Pavilion Publishing and Media Ltd.
Printing: CMP Digital Print Solutions

Contents

Acknowledgements

I would like to thank many people who in different ways supported and encouraged the writing of this book. Special thanks go to Sharon Cuthbert for nudging me to approach Pavilion in the first place. I would like to thank Mary Spence, Ros Leigh, Fiona Moorhouse, Noel Hess, Jeanne Magagna, Debbie Clarke and Sebastian Kraemer for encouraging my interest in maternal mental health as a 'second' career following my work in psychiatric rehabilitation.

Thanks also go to Jo Culham, Eleanor Grant, Mary-Ann Collis, Hannah Solemani, Gill Andrews, Carol Burtt, Abi Herbert, Sarah Lunn, the late Violet Gleeson, Anna Caffrey, Kathy Bonshor Evans, Andia Papadopoulou, Stella Balsamo, Cheryl Pelteret and Ros Wesson.

I should like to thank all my patients, whose resilience, courage, humour and honesty continue to inspire my thinking about motherhood and infancy. And also the generous and lovely family who allowed me to observe their firstborn as part of my Infant Observation Studies. Thanks also go to all the midwives and health visitors who have worked with me over the last 15 years and especially to Esther Boye and Bridie Newson who gave me such great examples of midwifery and health visitor care.

I am enormously grateful to my brilliant family. Firstly, my husband Phil, for his love and support of every kind throughout the writing of this book (and talking about it!). To my sons, Laurie and Linus, for their occasional I.T. assistance, but mostly for their refreshing pull towards everyday life. Also to Laurie for a few shared days researching in different reading rooms in the British Library.

Finally I would like to thank all my contributors; Eleanor Grant, Gemma Caton, Agnieszka Klimowicz, Elizabeth Best and Heather Jenkins, who made the writing of this book the multidisciplinary collaboration I knew it needed to be. Their warm and passionate enthusiasm for their work, and for sharing it in their writing, was a joyful part of the process.

Thanks also go to Kerry Boettcher, Ruth Chalmers and Kathleen Steeden at Pavilion Publishing.

Sue Gellhorn

About the authors

Elizabeth Best

Elizabeth is a consultant perinatal psychiatrist with the Medway and Swale mother and infant mental health service in Kent. She studied medicine at Sheffield University, and completed her postgraduate psychiatry training at the Maudsley, Guys and St Thomas' Hospitals. Her interest in perinatal mental health was encouraged in a post as a junior doctor with the Bethlem Royal Hospital mother and baby unit, and continued to develop in later posts as a specialist registrar with the MAPPIM perinatal mental health team at St Thomas's Hospital. Elizabeth is also accredited as a practitioner in cognitive analytic therapy.

As part of her current role, Elizabeth provides assessment and treatment for women with previous or current severe mental health difficulties, working collaboratively with them in the perinatal period, with their families and in liaison with other health professionals. She also regularly delivers teaching in perinatal mental health to a wide variety of health and social care professionals and trainees.

Gemma Caton

Gemma is a specialist health visitor in a parent infant mental health support service based in Great Yarmouth. She is employed by East Coast Community Health (CIC) NHS Trust but seconded by the Priory Children's Centre. She trained in Norfolk first as a paediatric nurse and then a health visitor. During her health visiting career that has so far spanned a decade she has received training in the CARE-Index, Mellow Parenting and the Solihull Parenting Approach. Interest in this field of work led to her completion of an MA in infant mental health from the Tavistock in London.

Her current role involves direct work with infants and their parents to promote a positive attachment relationship, and supervision and training of health visitors and children centre staff. She is particularly passionate about the Solihull Approach and the way it encourages health visitors and other professionals to think about the work with their clients.

Sue Gellhorn

Sue is a clinical psychologist with a long term interest in supporting and teaching front-line health practitioners. She worked for 28 years in adult mental health services in the NHS in London and Hertfordshire. Her first specialism was psychiatric rehabilitation, where she developed her interest in the application of psychodynamic understanding to the work of front-line care providers.

In the last 15 years she has worked in clinical, training and supervisory roles to support the mental health of women and babies in the perinatal period. Sue has provided training and supervision for health visitors working with postnatal depression, infant mental health and attachment across two boroughs in North London. From 2007 to 2012, she provided a specialist perinatal clinical service within the Islington Improved Access to Psychological Therapies (IAPT) service.

She has a small private clinical psychology practice in Islington, specialising in the treatment of women with perinatal mental health difficulties. Sue is currently training as a parent infant psychotherapist with Oxpip in Oxford.

Eleanor Grant

Eleanor is a clinical psychologist with 30 years' experience of working in the NHS in adult mental health. For 10 years she was consultant clinical psychologist with primary care psychological services in Great Yarmouth, Norfolk where she took a leading role in the development of maternal mental health services and promoting parent-infant support. She worked closely with local Sure Start centres as they developed and from 2002 to 2012 was a senior member of the clinical team at the Priory Sure Start Children's Centre, Great Yarmouth. During this time she helped produce the first integrated care pathway for maternal depression in Great Yarmouth and developed training, supervision and group work for the Parent Infant Mental Health Support (PIMHS) services at the Priory. She now works in independent practice.

Heather Jenkins

Heather is a specialist midwife for vulnerable adults and babies. She trained at King's College London and is now employed by Whittington Health NHS Trust in north London. Having worked as a midwife for 15 years, Heather has a wide variety of experience within the hospital and community settings and has worked closely with projects funded by Sure Start. Her current role involves providing specialist midwifery care to women with complex social needs and providing safeguarding supervision to midwives. Heather is a liaison midwife for the perinatal mental health team. She has a specialist interest in substance misuse and is currently involved in a research project with the University of Lancaster and Birth Companions charity. Heather is passionate about the midwives' role within perinatal mental health and raising the profile of midwives' training in this area.

Agnieszka Klimowicz

Agnieszka works as a consultant perinatal psychiatrist in Kent and holds a private practice in London.

She has a long-term interest in attachment theory and its application to mental health treatment particularly in the context of bonding difficulties and relationship problems.

She qualified as a doctor from the Jagiellonian University, Krakow, Poland, in 1996, trained both in psychiatry and psychotherapy, and was awarded a PhD for the dissertation: *Symptom versus personality changes after psychotherapy in patients with anxiety and somatization disorders.*

She is extensively involved in teaching medical students and trainees, as well as promoting perinatal and parental mental health.

Chapter 1: Introduction

Sue Gellhorn

This book is intended to be a helpful resource and source of inspiration for all midwives, health visitors, children's centre staff and others working to develop the care they can offer to women with maternal mental health difficulties and their babies. It is hoped that it may also be of use to GPs, obstetricians, practice nurses and other professionals providing psychological care in primary and maternity care settings.

All the contributors are passionate about maternal mental health and have a very strong commitment to training, teaching and supervising. Recent statements from the Department of Health (2015) and the professional bodies for midwifery and health visiting have noted that midwives and health visitors can feel ill-equipped and lacking in confidence to ask about and offer help with maternal mental health difficulties. Good training on perinatal mental health is only just beginning to shape up as service need is finally recognised. Many of the contributors have had to find their training and learning experiences on an ad hoc basis. Robust and comprehensive training in maternal mental health is not yet available for all those staff who need skills in this area. This means that providing care for women with mental health needs can feel like an isolated business. It is hoped this volume will serve as something similar to a knowledgeable and supportive colleague when challenging work provokes questions and doubt.

Mental health and the maternity journey

Having a baby is a powerful physical experience for a woman. It is also a powerful psychological experience, particularly for first time mothers, but also for women repeating the experience of childbirth at a different point in their lives.

Recent campaigns and national reports aimed at raising awareness (Bauer *et al*, 2014) have highlighted that the idea that little intervention is required in postnatal depression is very far from the case. Apart from the distress and psychological cost to mother and baby, the social and health costs of untreated perinatal mental health difficulties are huge. These include the costs of child and adolescent mental health services dealing with children's behavioural problems, special education provision, family courts, social services and probation services.

In the UK, maternity services, although at times overstretched, are well placed to provide physical and medical care to the pregnant woman in a variety of settings, including in her own home. However, services are now also becoming mindful of the psychological care or mental health support services a mother and baby may need in order to flourish, progress and enjoy life in the first year of parenting. Even more importantly for the new infant these are the formative experiences that will shape the foundation for the whole of their life. The NSPCC's *Prevention in Mind* report found that 122,000 babies under one were living with a parent who has a mental health problem (Hogg, 2013).

Whether her baby was planned or not, women come to motherhood with a personal history and a set of dreams and aspirations which affect the unfolding mother-baby relationship in two important ways. Firstly, they affect how the mother experiences her pregnancy, the events of giving birth and how she views herself as she begins to take on her role as mother. Secondly, they affect how she sees her baby, from the minute they are born to how she makes sense of their behaviour, cries and early infantile relating. These ideas of early mother-baby relationships will be explored in more depth in later chapters which will examine concepts such as attachment and 'mentalisation' (essentially the imagining of the mind of another) and how they shape the interplay of responses and connections between mothers and their babies (see Chapter 6).

When a mother is depressed, withdrawn or distressed by other psychological difficulties, if these issues are not picked up and attended to by others, her isolation and troubled state of mind may create a negative maternal journey. In another scenario, where a mother is making her best attempt at attentive and thoughtful care, but a good connection with the baby is lacking, then other sorts of help or treatment may be required. Of course there will be ups and downs in the journey of new motherhood, but ideally mistakes and bad days are balanced by a generally positive mother-baby connection. Caring for a baby involves a relationship, therefore providing professional care for these mothers and babies must involve building a relationship with both.

Postnatal depression is the best known, although not necessarily best understood, of the range of perinatal mental health difficulties. Recent research and developing clinical expertise have shown that it is important not to group all sorts of maternal mental health difficulties under this heading. For one thing, many women are known to experience a variety of mental health difficulties in pregnancy. For example, antenatal anxiety is now found to be extremely common and has a measureable impact on maternal and infant well-being. In addition, depression in the postnatal period has many differing presentations and without a knowledge base of the range of difficulties that can be experienced, misconceptions are likely, and help and treatment may not be accessed.

Case example: Catherine

Catherine was a successful lecturer in dance and theatre studies. She had always worked extremely hard to do well. She had a horror of acknowledging any personality traits which she saw as indicating 'weakness'. After the birth of her first baby she found the sleep deprivation and lack of structure to her day disorienting. She felt that she had lost sense of who she was and felt little connection to her new baby. For a few weeks she found it difficult to even communicate with her family and was unable to leave the house alone. Her GP diagnosed postnatal depression and recognised that she was quite unwell and in need of treatment and careful monitoring. A combination of GP support, medication and practical and emotional support from family helped her recover after a frightening couple of months.

Summary of key facts from NSPCC report *Prevention in Mind* (Hogg, 2013)

Maternal mental health difficulties are diverse and complex. With a better understanding of their nature midwives, GPs, obstetricians, health visitors and children's centre workers can work on prevention, identification and treatment of women to mitigate against the effects on families' and children's future well-being. This chimes with the Government recognition of 'no health without mental health' for real progress in public health (Department of Health, 2011).

Some women have no previous history of mental health difficulties prior to pregnancy and motherhood but for a number of reasons find the adjustment of lifestyle, relationships and the role that motherhood requires makes it difficult for them to cope. Other women may have a pre-existing mental illness which persists, deteriorates or recurs during the perinatal period. Women with schizophrenia and bipolar disorder are at a heightened risk of relapse of their illness when having a baby. Sadly, many women also avoid taking medication which has been keeping them well up until their pregnancy, often because they do not take advice about the best plan for their care and sometimes because they are ill-advised (see Chapter 9). Puerperal psychosis, which is much less common, is a very serious mental illness presenting risks to both mother and baby. The onset is typically within two weeks of the birth (and often in the first few days) and constitutes a psychiatric emergency.

Depression is especially common, with 10 to 14% of mothers affected either in pregnancy, postnatally or across their whole maternity experience. Tearfulness, feeling low, poor concentration, irritability and feeling overwhelmed are very common symptoms observed or reported by women. However anxiety is also now known to be very common, both in pregnancy and after giving birth. Anxiety often takes the form of excessive concern about the baby's well-being and after birth can lead to hypervigilance towards the baby and sometimes sleep difficulties as a result. Much of the focus in previous decades has been on depression but there is now better recognition of anxiety symptoms, both as part of the clinical picture in perinatal depression but also as part of other disorders, such as perinatal obsessive compulsive disorder and post-traumatic stress disorder (PTSD), and existing as a clinical problem in its own right.

PTSD appears to be more common in pregnant women than in the general population. Symptoms of earlier trauma can emerge at this time, especially for women who have experienced childhood abuse or sexual abuse. For these women, pregnancy, becoming a parent and the physical intimacy of delivery and baby care can create problems.

For many women there is a continuity in their symptoms from pregnancy to early motherhood and therefore there is scope for professionals to support and intervene early on in pregnancy to work on prevention. Indeed, for women who have been depressed earlier in their life, sometimes for several years, intervention when they become pregnant is especially important.

Taking the opportunity to offer mental health care

The frequency of health care contacts when women are pregnant or have just given birth presents good opportunities to offer services to women with mental health difficulties who may not have been diagnosed or offered treatment before. The first step is recognition and detection (see Chapter 3) facilitated by asking about psychological health and well-being. This can then be followed by listening, sensitive support and the offer of effective treatment approaches. Women also need to be kept in mind by the different parts of primary care and community services, so that women who do not take up or feel comfortable with what is first offered can be followed up and offered a different kind of service or treatment.

Babies' development and urgency in maternal mental health care

Help for perinatal mental health problems needs to be sensitive and prompt – a baby's development is unfolding day-by-day and their experience is minutely influenced by their mother's mood, sense of well-being and daily functioning.

Estimated numbers of women affected by perinatal
mental illnesses in England each year

1,380 Postpartum psychosis

Postpartum psychosis is a severe mental illness that typically affects
women in the weeks after giving birth, and causes symptoms such
as confusion, delusions, paranoia and hallucinations.

Rate: 2/1000 maternities

1,380 Chronic serious mental illness

Chronic serious mental illnesses are longstanding mental illnesses,
such as schizophrenia or bipolar disorder, which may be more likely
to develop, recur or deteriorate in the perinatal period.

Rate: 2/1000 maternities

20,640 Severe depressive illness

Severe depressive illness is the most serious form of depression,
where symptoms are severe and persistent, and significantly impair
a woman's ability to function normally.

Rate: 30/1000 maternities

20,640 Post traumatic stress disorder (PTSD)

PTSD is an anxiety disorder caused by very stressful, frightening or
distressing events, which may be relived through intrusive, recurrent
recollections, flashbacks and nightmares.

Rate: 30/1000 maternities

86,020 Mild to moderate depressive illness and
anxiety states

Mild-moderate depressive illness includes symptoms such as
persistent sadness, fatigue and a loss of interest and enjoyment in
activities. It often co-occurs with anxiety, which may be experienced
as distress, uncontrollable worries, panic or obsessive thoughts.

Rate: 100-150/1000 maternities

154,830 Adjustment disorders and distress

Adjustment disorders and distress occur when a woman is unable to
adjust or cope with an event such as pregnancy, birth or becoming a
parent. A woman with these conditions will exhibit a distress reaction
that lasts longer, or is more excessive than would normally be
expected, but does not significantly impair normal function.

Rate: 150-300/1000 maternities

* There may be some women who experience more than one of these conditions.
Source: Estimated using prevalence figures in guidance produced by the Joint Commissioning Panel for Mental
Health in 2012 and ONS data on live births in England in 2011.

**Figure 1.1: Estimated numbers of women affected by perinatal mental
illnesses in England each year. Reprinted with permission from Hogg S
(2013)** *Prevention in Mind. All Babies Count: Spotlight on perinatal mental
health.* **NSPCC.**

There are three key tasks for parents in the early months of caring for their baby.

1. To establish a secure attachment to their baby so that the baby can begin to learn about the world, themselves and how to relate to others with parental help reliably available.

2. To help the baby with emotional regulation. This means helping the baby recognise and manage the ups and downs of daily life and the range of emotional states.

3. Build up secure attachment by everyday sensitive and responsive care from parents, noticing and attending to their baby's needs (see Chapter 6).

Studies have shown that babies' emotional and cognitive development is adversely affected by care giving from a mother who is clinically depressed (Murray *et al*, 2010).

These effects are mediated in complex ways. The two main ways the developing infant is affected are:

1. A neurophysiological impact on the baby's developing nervous and endocrine system.

2. A psychosocial impact on an infant's learning about themselves and how they can relate to others through a good connection (or otherwise) with their mother.

Studies have shown that pregnant women experiencing significant depression or anxiety produce higher levels of the stress hormone cortisol (Glover *et al*, 2010). This cortisol crosses the placenta and affects the developing nervous system of the foetus both in terms of neural structure and physiology. Babies with this inheritance do not regulate stress and emotions well and may be primed to be anxious and jumpy or suppress their emotions if cortisol levels are excessive and too high to be regulated.

Taken together, studies of infant development and neurophysiological research show that stress in infants is real and may have a significant impact on their emotional regulation and resilience as they develop (Glover *et al*, 2010; Gerhardt, 2015). It is recognised that the severity and chronicity of the mother's difficulties will mediate the effects on her baby. Glover (2014) also points out that some of the early effects measured that were linked to postnatal depression might have been the result of anxiety in late pregnancy which is now known to impact on hyperactivity and attention difficulties seen in young children. Studies are just beginning to provide evidence that the maternal care provided continues to influence the developing neurophysiology of a baby after birth (Bergman, 2010). This is encouraging for intervention programmes where mothers are known to have been stressed or depressed in pregnancy.

Avoiding the catch-all label

In National Guidance (NICE, 2014; Hogg, 2013) use of the term 'postnatal depression' is cautioned against. This is for a number of reasons, some of them highlighting serious consequences which have emerged from reports examining maternal and infant deaths.

Firstly, the Centre for Maternal and Child Enquiries (Oates & Cantwell, 2011) report underlined how when the term postnatal depression is used, women's mental health difficulties in the perinatal period can easily be seen as less serious than they actually are, in terms of severity of disturbance and risk. Secondly, evidence has shown that where women's difficulties are incorrectly given this label, without careful assessment or diagnosis it can obscure the details of other symptoms or experiences she is actually having. For example, a woman may be beginning to have symptoms which indicate puerperal psychosis, believing she is not the mother of her child or that her child is threatened by malevolent forces. Or she may be suffering from PTSD and experiencing flashbacks, panic attacks and de-personalisation. These disorders are not the same as postnatal depression but may be misdiagnosed as such. These difficulties will have a different impact on the woman and her baby and the intervention required will be very different.

The third reason why using the term postnatal depression as a catch-all label for new mothers is advised against is that, where there is a lack of knowledge about perinatal mental health, it can be confused with the so-called 'baby blues'. The 'baby blues' is a period of low or changeable mood and tearfulness which is very common after giving birth and passes in two to five days. It therefore needs little attention or intervention apart from reassurance that it is very common and will pass. This is not the case for many maternal mental health difficulties inappropriately referred to under the umbrella term 'postnatal depression'.

Overview of content and contributors

The book is a collaborative effort and has brought together multidisciplinary expertise from clinical psychology, midwifery, health visiting and perinatal psychiatry. All the contributors have an interest in excellent mental health service provision. They also have an interest in attachment and psychoanalytic ideas and especially care that thoughtfully acknowledges women and their individual stories.

Chapter 1: Introduction (by Sue Gellhorn)
This chapter has introduced postnatal depression and the spectrum of maternal mental health difficulties that women can experience across their maternity

journey. Key facts from the epidemiology of maternal mental health in the UK have been presented. The opportunities for offering mental health support and the crucial timeliness of this, in terms of protecting infant emotional development, have also been highlighted.

Chapter 2: Perspectives on postnatal depression (by Sue Gellhorn)
This chapter outlines how the understanding of maternal mental health has evolved over the past few decades and how it is conceptualised by different professional groups and academic specialties. How some of this thinking continues to inform our current understanding of women's difficulties and service provision in the area is examined.

Chapter 3: Detection, recognition and assessment of maternal mental health difficulties (by Sue Gellhorn)
This chapter examines the approaches and tools that are currently available for the detection and assessment of maternal mental health difficulties. Some of the barriers to the detection and recognition of these difficulties, for both professionals and the women themselves, are considered.

Chapter 4: Levels of intervention, treatment and support (by Sue Gellhorn)
This chapter looks at the levels of intervention, support and treatment that may be needed and the community, psychological and medical treatments that are typically offered in the UK at the time of writing. The national and professional guidance on treatment recommendations are considered.

Chapter 5: Normal anxieties in early motherhood and those needing professional attention (by Sue Gellhorn)
This chapter presents some of the common worries encountered in new mothers. Understanding the roots of some of these worries is explored. The chapter goes on to examine when pregnant women and mothers who are expressing worries to professionals might need further professional intervention. The vulnerability factors for postnatal depression are discussed.

Chapter 6: Keeping the baby in mind: baby-mindedness in parents and professionals (by Eleanor Grant)
This chapter introduces the concept of a mother's attachment to her infant and the impact of postnatal depression on this attachment. The theoretical understanding of maternal mental health difficulties from the perspective of a woman's own parenting and attachment history are considered. New clinical services which aim to support attachment relationships between mothers and their newborn infants are introduced.

Chapter 7: Working with the whole family (by Sue Gellhorn)
This chapter examines the impact of maternal mental health difficulties on the wider family. Working with fathers and partners in ante-natal preparation and postnatally, and supporting family members in different family contexts are considered. Cultural factors in different family situations are discussed.

Chapter 8: Supporting mothers in complex family contexts (by Sue Gellhorn)
This chapter examines the challenges of supporting pregnant women and new mothers approaching childbearing and parenting in complex family contexts. Providing care for asylum seekers and refugee families and supporting mothers and babies who are homeless are considered. Ways of working with mothers experiencing domestic violence and drug and alcohol addictions are also introduced.

Chapter 9: Severe perinatal mental health difficulties (by Agnieszka Klimowicz and Elizabeth Best)
This chapter gives key information about the less common but more severe perinatal mental illnesses, including postpartum psychosis and severe postnatal depression. The learning points from the CMACE (2011) enquiries are highlighted. The role of perinatal psychiatry services and mother and baby units and of midwives and health visitors in liaising with these services is described.

Chapter 10: Other types of maternal mental health difficulties (by Sue Gellhorn)
This chapter considers a number of common maternal mental health difficulties which need to be understood as distinct from postnatal depression, but may also be found as co-morbid conditions alongside postnatal depression. These include obsessive compulsive disorder, anxiety disorders, post-traumatic stress disorder and personality disorder.

Chapter 11: Challenges for midwives (by Heather Jenkins)
This chapter considers the particular challenges for midwives and maternity services in providing care for women with maternal mental health difficulties. The challenges of having sensitive conversations with women where continuity of care is compromised are examined. Training and organisational issues for midwives are considered. The role of supporting women taking medication and making decisions about medication and breastfeeding is covered.

Chapter 12: Challenges for health visitors (by Gemma Caton)
This chapter explores the variety of roles taken up by health visitors in relation to maternal mental health. The opportunities provided by an ongoing relationship with young families are highlighted. The theoretical concepts underpinning

listening visits and new mother-baby interventions are discussed, and organisational challenges for the health visiting profession are presented.

Chapter 13: Perinatal mental health pathways and networks (by Eleanor Grant and Gemma Caton)
This chapter looks at how to make care pathways for maternal mental health a reality. National and professional developments focusing on improving care pathways are highlighted. Making good professional links and referrals to other community and expert providers is considered. The development and role of local service champions are discussed. The importance of clinical supervision and self-care for professionals working with mothers and babies in difficulty is emphasised.

References

Bauer A, Parsonage M, Knapp M, Lemmi V & Adelaja B (2014) *The Costs of Perinatal Mental Health Problems* [online]. PSSRU and the Centre for Mental Health. Available at: http://eprints.lse.ac.uk/59885/ (accessed April 2016).

Bergman K, Sarkar P, Glover V & O'Connor T (2010) Maternal prenatal cortisol and infant cognitive development: moderation by infant-mother attachment. *Biological Psychiatry* **67** (11) 1026–1032.

Centre for Maternal and Child Enquiries (CMACE) (2011) Saving mothers' lives: reviewing maternal deaths to make motherhood safer. *British Journal of Obstetrics and Gynaecology* **118** (S1) 1–203.

Department of Health (2011) *No Health without Mental Health: A cross-government mental health outcomes strategy for people of all ages* [online]. Available at: www.mhpf.org.uk/sites/default/files/documents/publications/dh_124058.pdf (accessed April 2016).

Department of Health (2015) *Improving Access to Perinatal Mental Health Services in England – A review*. Available at: http://www.nhsiq.nhs.uk/media/2696378/nhsiq_perinatal_mental_health_sml__0915final.pdf (accessed April 2016).

Gerhardt S (2015) *Why Love Matters: How affection shapes a baby's brain*. Hove: Routledge.

Glover V (2014) Maternal depression, anxiety and stress during pregnancy and child outcome: what needs to be done. *Clinical Obstetrics Gynaecology* **28** (1) 25–35.

Glover V, O'Connor TG & O'Donnell K (2010) Prenatal stress and the programming of the HPA axis. *Neuroscience and Behavioural Reviews* **35** (1) 17–22.

Hogg S (2013) *Prevention in Mind. All Babies Count: Spotlight on perinatal mental health* [online]. NSPCC. Available at: http://everyonesbusiness.org.uk/wp-content/uploads/2014/06/NSPCC-Spotlight-report-on-Perinatal-Mental-Health.pdf (accessed April 2016).

Murray l, Halligan S & Cooper P (2010) Effects of postnatal depression on mother-infant interactions and child development. In: JG Bremner and TD Wachs (Eds) *Handbook of Infant Development, Vol.2* (2nd edition). Oxford: Wiley Blackwell.

NICE (2014) *Antenatal and Postnatal Mental Health: Clinical management and service guidance* [online]. Available at: https://www.nice.org.uk/guidance/cg192 (accessed April 2016).

Oates M & Cantwell R (2011) Deaths from psychiatric causes. In: Centre for Maternal and Child Enquiries (CMACE) Saving Mothers' Lives: Reviewing Maternal Deaths To Make Motherhood Safer: 2006-08. *BJOG* **118** (S1) 1–203.

Chapter 2: Perspectives on postnatal depression

Sue Gellhorn

Perinatal mental health difficulties, especially postnatal depression, have been viewed and studied in different fields and with differing emphasis over the last four decades. This chapter will look at these various perspectives on depression in new mothers.

Biological psychiatry

The approach of biological psychiatry is to employ a medical disease model where symptoms of mental ill health are seen as a reflection of a biological disorder. In the case of postnatal depression, this was originally seen as developing as a result of the very marked hormonal changes present in pregnancy, labour and immediately post-delivery. This approach is characterised by the work of Dalton (1980). For some women hormonal factors do seem implicated in considerable emotional turmoil. As in premenstrual tension, for some new mothers there was seen to be an apparent link between extreme hormonal fluctuations and changes in mood. This biological view led to treatment with hormone-based physical treatments in the past. However, while antidepressants (which work on the physiological system of neurotransmitters) may be used in the treatment of many women with depression after giving birth, the testing of hormone levels and treatment with hormone supplements is relatively uncommon in current practice.

Feminist perspectives and community psychology

The idea that struggling with depression alongside the care of a newborn is a result of a structuring of society that minimises women's tasks and workload, and hence their need for any additional practical help and emotional support, has had a lot of support since the 1970s and still makes sense in 2016. Researchers like sociologist Anne Oakley (1980) have highlighted the invisibility of some of women's burdens, particularly those raising children in poverty or as single parents, but also better off women who are isolated due to a partner who works very long hours or travels for work.

Community psychology interventions, which see the importance of avoiding pathologising individuals and reduce mental distress through social action at a community level, were the pre-cursor of current services developed through Sure Start (a UK Government initiative) and are now embodied in local children's centres. In the 1980s, the Bridge Project in White City, west London, set up by psychotherapist Sue Holland, recognised that the benefits of individual therapy could be more helpfully delivered via a different model for women living in large, multi-ethnic council estates (Holland, 1994) (see also Chapter 4). Similarly the Newpin projects, developed by Andrea Pound in the 1970s, offered professional and social support to women experiencing postnatal depression, understanding that their depression was partly a reflection of the role and low status of motherhood in urban Western communities (Pound & Abel, 1996).

Social psychiatry

The pioneering and thoughtful work of a sociologist and a psychotherapist Brown and Harris (1978) has become one of the foundations of modern day social psychiatry and current public health thinking about well-being in different communities and populations. Brown and Harris collected a great deal of data about women with different degrees of depression in Camberwell in south London. They delineated three key aspects of depression which are particularly relevant to depression in the perinatal period. Brown and Harris are well known for their development of ideas about life events in the aetiology of mental distress and illness, but they also uncovered how important changes in thinking about the world and the self are for an individual who is succumbing to depression and a depressed outlook on life.

They came to understand that both external events, for example having a third baby or the lift in your block of flats breaking down, and internal world events, for example believing that you are a bad mother or having thoughts that you do not love your baby like a real mother should, will both have a role in contributing to the likelihood of depression.

Furthermore, from an epidemiological point of view, the key findings were that women with several young children under school age were more likely to be depressed than those without, and sadly, they were also less likely to be consulting their GP for help with these difficulties. Another very important finding was that women with someone to confide in about their life and their difficulties, especially a husband or partner, were less likely to be depressed. This has come to be seen as one of the most protective factors in relation to developing mental illness and is central to present day ideas about good 'mental well-being'. Brown and Harris' work involved very time consuming surveys listening to women in detail and over time (i.e. longitudinal studies) talking about their experiences, stories and their histories. This gave key insights into the experience of women with perinatal mental difficulties and was very helpful in understanding what may help in terms of support and treatment.

Case example: Selen

Selen is a young Turkish woman who struggled in pregnancy with severe back pain. She comes from a family of five where her violent father had always been protected by the family's shame and solidarity over his violence. Selen finally left home when an attack from her father left her with a painful injury to her back. At the time of her pregnancy, Selen's father was seriously ill with cancer and her family wanted her to forgive him and resume contact with him. Her conflict with her female relatives for putting her under this pressure left her depressed, angry and isolated from family support. She experienced chronic pain and her loving and sensitive husband found it impossible to help her look forward to the birth of their first child. Selen was critical of the doctors and midwives who she felt did not understand how much her pain affected her.

In summary, Brown and Harris (1978) found that:

- Social factors, such as financial stresses, housing problems and noisy or aggressive neighbours can contribute to the development of depression.

- Negative views and judgements about the self contribute to feelings of depression.

- Early childhood experience, especially the loss of a parent before the age of 11 and neglectful or abusive parenting, increases the likelihood of depression in adulthood.

- Women with access to a supportive partner or other confiding relationship (such as a mother, sister or a close friend) are less likely to become depressed than women who don't.

This last point is the basis of many first level interventions for perinatal mental health difficulties. For example, listening visits, which may be provided by health visitors and family nurses, provide the same empathic support and containment of anxiety that more fortunate women may be able to access from their own social network. All four points together are very helpful to bear in mind when offering help to women and planning care pathways and services to support them.

The psychosocial model of postnatal depression

The major contribution of the psychosocial model of postnatal mental health disorders is that we are clear that adverse life events and stress can contribute to the onset of depression. But in terms of care giving, it is also clear that support of various kinds can ameliorate these difficulties. It furthers our understanding of individual women's difficulties to look in detail at the normal stresses of motherhood. That is to say the stresses that impinge on all women having a baby, and particularly a first baby.

The normal stresses of motherhood

- Sleep deprivation.
- Being faced with a lot of repetitive tasks and simultaneous demands.
- Being responsible for a baby's welfare and survival.
- Loss of former (work) role and former social network.
- Time with her partner interrupted.
- Less income and little or no independent income.
- Difficulty expressing dissatisfaction with motherhood.
- Pressure of society's ideals of motherhood and parenthood.
- Unrealistic expectations of herself as a mother.
- Pressure to return to the workplace.

For women with perinatal mental health difficulties, many of these pressures will be present, but in the context of ongoing mental health difficulties. For such women additional help, support and treatment will usually be needed to support good outcomes for mother and baby.

A psychoanalytic perspective

Although psychoanalysts and child psychotherapists have shown interest in depression and in understanding infants and infantile experiences, there has been surprisingly little interest in examining the psychodynamic processes at work in women who are suffering from postnatal depression. Notable exceptions are Joan Raphael-Leff (2009) who presents a description of women's psychological approaches to motherhood as either 'facilitators' or 'regulators'. Rozsika Parker

(2005) also takes a very detailed look at the stresses and conflicts inherent in maternal ambivalence; essentially women's love-hate relationship with their demanding new role.

Lawrence Blum (2007), however, gives a very useful account of three key conflicts which were often at play in women he has seen in his clinical practice. These concepts will make a lot of sense to anyone who has spent time talking to new mothers in difficulty and can be very helpful in helping them and professionals make sense of what has gone wrong.

These conflicts are:

- a conflict about dependency
- a conflict about expressing anger
- a difficult identification with their own mother.

Dependency conflicts

Despite our Western emphasis on independence, we can all have a wish to be cared for and enjoy a dependent state. This rapidly gets pushed aside as we can see in the childhood taunt, 'you big baby!'. However all new mothers need a certain amount of looking after as was well recognised in the early 20th century maternity homes where a two week stay for nursing mothers was expected. Early motherhood can stir up all sorts of feelings of dependency as a new mother struggles to meet all the 24 hour demands of her newborn. As Blum says:

'If she can accept her dependent needs and ensure that she is in fact taken care of, and if she can tolerate her baby's dependency and her reactions to it, she is unlikely to develop postpartum depression. If she cannot, she may be at risk.'
(Blum, 2007)

Anger conflicts

It is common for women with postnatal depression to have problems with feelings of anger. Mothers typically feel they do not have any justification to feel angry (especially if they have been trying for a baby for a long time), they feel guilty about having angry feelings and they are frightened to express any anger. However motherhood brings many stresses, short-term losses and frustrations. If a new mother can acknowledge and use these stresses as a prompt to get herself some extra help or time for herself, she will be able to manage. If she isn't able to do so, feelings can escalate and may result in obsessional thoughts about the baby coming to harm (see Chapter 9) or impulsive loss of control.

Motherhood conflicts

It is common for women with postnatal depression to report difficult relationships with their own mother. They may feel that they do not want to repeat the experience they had, which they feel was not sensitive and loving. However, providing tender loving care when you are feeling deprived yourself and do not have an internal model of what this is like to draw on, is difficult. Women with this sort of history find the everyday judgements of how much to give and when to say no very difficult.

We can see that the many areas of study, research and theorising can help us bring a thoughtful open-mindedness to the women and babies we are trying to help and offer treatment. But the more we are able to take time to talk to them and really listen to their experience as they try and make sense of it themselves, the more likely we are likely to be in a position to offer real help.

References

Blum LD (2007) Psychodynamics of postpartum depression. *Psychoanalytic Psychology* **24** (1) 45–62.

Brown GW & Harris T (1978) *Social Origins of Depression: A study of psychiatric disorder in women*. Abingdon: Tavistock Publications.

Dalton K (1980) *Depression After Childbirth*. Oxford: Oxford University Press.

Holland S (1994) From social abuse to social action: A neighbourhood psychotherapy and social action project for women. In J Ussher and P Nicholson (Eds) *Gender Issues in Clinical Psychology*. London: Routledge.

Oakley A (1980) *Women Confined: Towards a sociology of childbirth*. Oxford: Martin Robertson.

Parker R (2005) *Torn in Two: The experience of maternal ambivalence*. London: Virago.

Pound A & Abel K (1996) Motherhood and mental illness. In: K Abel, M Buszewicz, S Davison, S Johnson and E Staples (Eds) *Planning Community Mental Health Services for Women*. London: Routledge.

Raphael-Leff J (2009) *Psychological Processes of Childbearing* (4th edition). London: Anna Feud Centre.

Chapter 3: Detection, recognition and assessment of maternal mental health difficulties

Sue Gellhorn

Medical assessment and monitoring of pregnancy and the newborn has been extended enormously over the past two or three decades. Antenatal screening programmes and newborn health checks can reveal a great deal more about the health of a mother, foetus or infant than was possible in previous generations.

However, the detection strategies, interventions and technologies associated with addressing the emotional health of mothers and babies are more challenging than those in the field of physical health. This is primarily because at all stages the assessment work and health contacts in this domain involve having a conversation. Some of these conversations are inevitably tentative, or searching, or need to be undertaken between a number of contacts, but the health assessments needed require a dialogue between a health worker and the mother, often about difficult feelings, thoughts or experiences. These experiences might be, for example, to do with alcohol problems, domestic violence, anxiety about childbirth or previous difficulties with obsessional symptoms such as excessive checking and cleaning.

The aim of this chapter is to examine the settings, tools and approaches that can be employed to undertake this work. Wherever professionals and community workers are coming into contact with pregnant women and mothers and babies, keeping an eye out for maternal mental health difficulties is important. The approach each worker takes will depend on local policy, professional practice guidelines and the settings where health contacts are taking place.

Maternal and infant mental health is a field that is getting increasing attention and if serious cases are missed, the outcomes can be very tragic. This fact, highlighted by the Centre for Maternal and Child Enquiries (Oates & Cantwell,

2011) which reports every three years, means that concern and anxiety is being generated in organisations and services which have responsibilities to provide care. Their staff are required to make assessments and referrals for specialist input and make judgements about risk and safeguarding. This can result in an over-emphasis on systems and procedure which can, in turn, create anxiety in professionals on the ground to 'follow protocol' and a tendency to focus on the administrative process at the expense of building trust with the women and mothers they are hoping to attend to.

The emphasis in this chapter will be on creating opportunities for sensitive conversations at appropriate times. Local care pathways vary but the national and professional guidance that currently exists will be highlighted and the implications for everyday practice discussed.

Common barriers to recognition and detection of postnatal depression

Depression postnatally is often overlooked and there are a number of factors contributing to this. Part of the aim of this book is to minimise this oversight and that with the readers' careful assessment and thoughtful professional input, mothers and babies in difficulty will be more likely to get help.

Some of the factors that get in the way of recognition and detection of depression at this stage of life are presented below.

- **Heterogeneous presentations**
  Symptoms or changes in behaviour are not those expected or thought of as typical of depression. For example women presenting with irritability and snappiness, rather than tearfulness and feelings of sadness.

- **Stigma of mental health difficulties**
  The stigma that still exists, despite societal shifts in the right direction, about having emotional or psychological difficulties – especially when they come at the same time as becoming a parent.

- **Cultural expectations**
  In a number of faiths a baby is considered a gift from God, so women, even if able to identify depressive feelings in themselves, feel that it would be culturally unacceptable to express them and they themselves would feel in conflict with their own faith to fully acknowledge them.

- **Presenting a brave front**
  Many women, especially those who have previously been successful in the workplace or who have particularly cherished the idea of motherhood, can make

a huge effort to mask their depression. They dress well, apply make-up and keep everything that is on show clean and organised, while feeling desperate inside and unable to cope or know what they should be doing for themselves and their baby.

■ **Depression and social context**

A mistaken belief that postnatal depression is only about difficulties to do with the baby or giving birth. Mothers struggling with social problems like poor housing, overcrowding or noisy neighbours can be missed. A health visitor or children's centre worker may say, 'I don't think this mother has postnatal depression it's just her housing problem'. The mother may indeed be depressed because of the social and practical circumstances in which she is raising her baby. These circumstances increase the everyday burden of care, especially if she has little support or help with problem solving around these difficulties. As with any depression, sorting out problems and prioritising is very difficult when you are feeling depressed.

Case example: Tasha

Following a difficult childhood when Tasha felt that her parents had always been pre-occupied with running their business, she had a serious relationship with a man who was 10 years older. Soon after medical investigations for some worrying symptoms, he died suddenly of a brain haemorrhage when Tasha was 22. She had been with him when he died and for some time afterwards often relived the events of the day of his death. A few years later she was in a new relationship with a loving and supportive partner and they were expecting their first child. However, from the beginning of the pregnancy, she found it difficult to manage her anxieties about the baby and found the contact with hospitals and health professionals distressing. At her booking appointment with a midwife, she felt able to say she was 'a worrier'. With sensitive questioning, her midwife recognised that she was probably suffering from an anxiety disorder, possibly PTSD relating to the events of her first partner's death. Without rushing to pass her on to another professional, they were able to start to explore the sources of help that might improve her mental well-being throughout the pregnancy and as she prepared for the birth.

Assessment and detection of ante-natal and postnatal anxiety

As discussed in Chapter 1, there is now much better recognition that anxiety is a common feature of pregnancy and new motherhood. However, to date there has been much less emphasis on developing specific tools to help with the assessment of anxiety. Because the research literature and clinical practice is only just catching up with women's difficulties in this area, this chapter inevitably covers more assessment tools that are concerned with the symptoms of depression.

Assessment tools

All primary healthcare providers and midwifery staff are trained to carry out a general assessment of health and functioning including emotional well-being and mental health. This section is intended to help health professionals extend this assessment to the detection of postnatal depression and other mental health difficulties with the help of assessment tools. The important point to remember is that these tools are not a replacement for a professional clinical assessment. In all cases, the best approach is to make use of any assessment tool in the context of a thoughtful conversation.

Various tools for the assessment of postnatal depression and maternal mental health problems have been developed for several purposes; research studies, identifying mental health needs in whole populations of mothers and in individual women. The constraints, cost benefits and the nature of the task are very different in these three contexts. However it is interesting to note that the same tools have often been used in all three scenarios. The Edinburgh Postnatal Depression Scale (EPDS) in particular is very often used for all three purposes.

The main assessment tools that will be considered in this chapter are:

- the EPDS
- the Whooley questions
- the Hospital Anxiety and Depression Scale (HADS) and the Patient Health Questionnaire (PHQ-9)
- the Community Practitioners and Health Visitors Association (CPHVA) 'How are you feeling?' booklets
- the antenatal and postnatal promotional guides
- the Wellbeing Plan
- a suggested interview structure for Maternal Mental Health Assessment.

1. The EPDS

The EPDS is the most well known and historically the most widely used assessment tool. It has been used extensively in research into postnatal depression in Britain and many other parts of the world. It is a 10 item self-report questionnaire developed in Edinburgh by clinicians looking for a practical measure to 'screen' new mothers for the presence of depression in community health care settings (Cox *et al*, 1987). It was designed to improve on scales such as the Beck Depression Inventory (BDI) (Beck *et al*, 1961) which were felt to distort scores because of their inclusion of somatic items such as tiredness, which were present in all new mothers whether they were depressed or not. Because it includes items covering a variety of experiences and symptoms that a new mother may be having, it is a very useful tool for opening up a conversation with a woman about her current experience.

There has been confusion about a number of ideas related to assessment, detection, screening and diagnosis in relation to the way the EPDS has been used. In more recent times it has received criticism for its medical model foundations and its misuse in pressured clinic settings where it has been reduced to a tick-box exercise by time-poor care providers and risk-averse service managers. All the current research shows that women find this type of approach particularly unhelpful and it discourages women from placing trust in their service providers and asking for further help (Coyle & Adams, 2002; Shakespeare *et al*, 2003).

Despite its use in research and clinical settings the EPDS is really designed to be used by health practitioners, such as health visitors, with the expectation of a face-to-face discussion about feelings and symptoms.

The EPDS has been a very successful tool. Much of what is known about maternal mental health difficulties outside of the UK was initially facilitated by the use of the EPDS in cross-cultural studies. In the 1980s and 1990s much work on detection and early intervention was carried out in the UK, especially within health visiting teams. In the best practice models, health visiting teams received comprehensive training on understanding postnatal depression, the use of the EPDS and training to offer first level talking treatment in the form of listening visits. The strongest evidence for the clinical efficacy of detection programmes for postnatal depression using the EPDS comes from clinical research trials where postnatal screening strategies were integrated with ongoing clinical management strategies provided by trained health professionals (Howard *et al*, 2014; Morrell *et al*, 2009).

Population screening for postnatal depression

The use of the EPDS as a screening tool to look for perinatal depression across whole populations is controversial (Milgrom *et al*, 2011). In the UK the current recommendation by the National Screening Committee (NSC) is that systematic population screening is not recommended (Hill, 2010). The criteria to be met for the implementation of whole population screening for a disorder include:

- The condition should be an important health problem.

- There should be a simple, safe, precise and validated screening test.

- There should be agreed evidence-based policies covering which individuals should be offered treatment and the appropriate treatment to be offered.

- Adequate staffing and facilities for testing, diagnosis, treatment and programme management should be available prior to the commencement of the screening programme.

The screening committee assessed that there was insufficient evidence to support the implementation of whole population screening for postnatal depression in the UK. This is in contrast, for example, with antenatal physical health screening for human immunodeficiency virus (HIV) in pregnant women, which continues to be recommended. However, part of the problem is that good intervention programmes, treatment and support are still not universally provided. In addition, the question of what works for whom is complex in mental health, and means that meeting NSC criteria concerning treatment is challenging.

As a result, whole population screening using the EPDS is not recommended, but its use as part of a comprehensive clinical assessment is. The use of the EPDS as part of an initial assessment with women fits well with the overall approach to maternal mental health within public health. The health visitor programme outlines the level of service offered as part of 'universal services' (all pregnant women, mothers and families) and that which is offered at the level called 'universal plus'. This fits with the idea of an initial high sensitivity 'screen', followed up with a more in depth assessment and discussion if indicated.

Maternal mental health work comes into the 'universal plus' service level for health visiting services. Within the 'universal plus' programme all women identified with a mild to moderate mental health issue need to be offered a range of support from well-being advice to medication and baby massage (see Chapter 4 on interventions).

Clinical assessment incorporating the EPDS

The EPDS is a 'paper and pencil' screening questionnaire which can be used in universal services to ask a woman about her mental health. It comprises 10 questions about how she has felt over the previous week. The scale is best administered by a health professional who has been trained in its use and can use it as a basis for opening up a discussion about how the woman is coping and how she has been feeling. Because it covers more than a very brief screen, the EPDS is particularly useful in opening up a conversation about mental well-being and indicating to women that her health professional is interested in her mood both now and in the future.

Each item on the scale carries a score of 0-3 giving a maximum score of 30. The EPDS indicates symptoms that may suggest current depression and elements of anxiety. In most identification programmes in universal services, a cut-off of 12 and above is used as indicative of the possible presence of depression and the need for a follow-up assessment. As with all assessment tools, there will be some false positives (women identified as possibly affected by depression who are not in fact depressed) and false negatives (women who are depressed but who are not identified by the assessment tool). Initially the EPDS was used at a six week postnatal check, but as postnatal depression often develops after this period it is very helpful for it to be repeated at two further time points postnatally.

The EPDS is recommended to support the clinical assessment of pregnant women and mothers in the following professional guidance:

- *Specialist Mental Health Midwives: what they do and why they matter* (Maternal Mental Health Alliance, 2013). This briefing makes recommendations to midwives about identifying risk and assessing current well-being. It recommends discussing and documenting details of women's past and current mental health, and looking out for any indicators that this may be deteriorating. They suggest midwives can use the EPDS as part of their clinical assessment.

- The Institute of Health Visiting (IHV) recommends that health visitors routinely assess for signs of mental health problems using brief screening questions. They emphasise that this questioning must be supported by the use of clinical skills such as observation, listening and paraphrasing to come to a clinical judgement. They recommend further assessment using a tool such as the EPDS which was specifically developed for use in primary care by health visitors (IHV, 2014).

- The timeline for assessment recommended in the Department of Health guidance document (Department of Health, 2012) for maternal mental health is postnatal reviews at 6-8 weeks, 3-4 months and 8-12 months.

■ NICE Guidance – *Antenatal and Postnatal Mental Health* (2014). NICE guidance from December 2014 recommends initial questioning about a woman's mental health and well-being using two brief depression identification questions (see the Whooley questions below). It then recommends that, where a positive mental health concern is detected, the worker considers following this up with a fuller assessment using the EPDS or the PHQ-9.

The key elements of successful protocols using the EPDS as part of maternal mental health assessment are:

■ effective training of all staff using the tool

■ using the scale as part of a face-to-face clinical interview at a home visit or in a place providing quiet privacy in a clinic or community centre

■ front line staff have good knowledge of local treatment, support services and referral pathways

■ staff undertaking assessments have good access to local mental health specialists, preferably for regular supervision of their maternal mental health work or, at the least, for consultation and advice.

All these points are emphasised in the new *National Framework for Continuing Professional Development for Health Visitors* (IHV, 2015)

2. The Whooley Questions

The Whooley questions are two to three 'screening' questions which are briefer and less time consuming to ask or administer than the EPDS. The tool was developed with an eye on utility in terms of the costs of health professionals' time and a cost-benefit analysis of different tools.

In the 2007 NICE guidance for antenatal and postnatal mental health there was a firm recommendation for health practitioners to assess for maternal mental health difficulties at each health contact from the midwife's booking visit to the 8-12 month postnatal contact with health visitors at a children's centre or health centre. In the revised guideline (NICE, 2014) this recommendation is retained, with the recommended tool being the Whooley questions.

'Recognising mental health problems in pregnancy and the postnatal period and referral.

At a woman's first contact with primary care or her booking visit, and during the early postnatal period, consider asking the following depression identification questions as part of a general discussion about a woman's mental health and wellbeing:

- *During the past month, have you often been bothered by feeling down, depressed, or hopeless?*

- *During the past month, have you often been bothered by little interest or pleasure in doing things?'*

(NICE, 2014)

However, the Whooley questions were originally validated on a single sex clinic population of older men in San Francisco (Whooley *et al*, 1997). Following misgivings about recommendations for a tool which had not been validated or used extensively with women and particularly women in the perinatal period, Mann *et al* (2012) undertook a study to validate the case-finding questions with a perinatal population of women in Bradford, UK. The women were receiving either ante or postnatal care in NHS services. This study validated the questions against the so-called 'gold standard' psychiatric diagnosis as determined via a structured clinical interview for Diagnostic and Statistical Manual, 4th Edition (DSM-IV) over the telephone.

Mann *et al*'s findings support the utility of the Whooley questions with a perinatal population and point out that the brevity of the case-finding questions save professionals significant amounts of time. In their view the ability to rule out depression would help to substantially reduce the number of women needing a more extensive assessment of their antenatal and postnatal mental health needs. There are both gains and losses with its brevity. It is perhaps useful in enabling professionals to decide who to spend more time on within a very large caseload, but its brevity also gives women little opportunity to open up about any difficulties they may be having. The Boots Family Trust survey identified that women were often not aware that their mental well-being was being assessed and midwives felt that the questions were too brief with the concern that more women with difficulties were being missed (Boots Family Trust Alliance 2013a).

The use of the Whooley questions is recommended by:

- NICE (2014) guidelines (as above). They recommend that at a first contact with primary care or maternity booking visit, and during the early postnatal period, the professional considers asking the Whooley (depression identification) questions as part of a general discussion about a women's mental health and well-being.

- The Maternal Mental Health Alliance (2013) emphasise the valuable role of all midwives in improving perinatal mental health. In terms of identifying risk and current well-being they suggest midwives can use tools such as the Whooley questions to strengthen their skilled clinical assessment.

- The Institute of Health Visiting (IHV, 2014) recommends the use of the Whooley tool for initial questions and that any response indicative of difficulties should be followed up using the EPDS or PHQ-9 (see page 33).They emphasise that all tools can produce both false positives and negatives and that the clinical assessment and judgement of the practitioner is key.

3. The Hospital Anxiety and Depression Scale (HADS)

The Hospital Anxiety and Depression Scale (HADS) was developed by Zigmond and Snaith (1983). It is a self-assessment scale developed to detect anxiety and depressive states in the general population. It comprises 14 statements about experiences over the past week. Seven items pertain to anxiety, worry and difficulty relaxing. The remaining seven items examine areas such as appearance, ability to concentrate and general feelings of happiness. The advantage of using this tool with the perinatal population is that it is looking to pick up signs of anxiety as well as depression, which other tools such as the EPDS do not cover well. A Boots Family Trust survey found that 12% of professionals were using the HADS to assess current emotional state. This group of professionals were mostly family nurse practitioners (Boots Family Trust Alliance, 2013a).

The HADS is recommended in *The Maternal Mental Health Pathway* (Department of Health, 2012).

In pregnancy

The Department of Health guidance recommends that the HADS may be used by midwives as a follow on from the Whooley questions at a booking appointment around 8-12 weeks of pregnancy.

At 32-36 weeks, the guidance recommends that all women are reviewed in terms of mental well-being using the Whooley questions and a supplementary mental health assessment is carried out using the HADS or the EPDS if there is an indication of mental distress.

Postnatally (birth visit to 10-14 days)

The Department of Health guidance recommends that the midwife updates the health visitor on the health, emotional and social status of both mother and baby. It also recommends that the midwife asks the NICE recommended questions (Whooley) if the woman's previous responses were 'no'. This is because evidence from audits shows that women are more likely to disclose mental health difficulties with repeated asking.

This maternal mental health assessment might take place in the obstetric or midwifery unit, the woman's home or local children's centre. At the new birth visit (health visitor) and 6-8 weeks, 3-4 months and 8-12 months the guidance recommends that the health visitor carries out a comprehensive assessment of the physical and emotional health of mother and baby. The assessment should include the Whooley questions and clinical judgement to assess maternal mood. Supplementary mental health assessments such as the HADS or the EPDS may also be used.

This pathway focuses on the role of the health visitor but also recognises the essential contributions of health provider partners in midwifery, mental health, general practice and third sector services (Department of Health, 2012).

4. The Patient Health Questionnaire (PHQ-9)

This self-report questionnaire has content based directly on the diagnostic criteria for a major depressive disorder as defined in the DSM-IV. As such, it is frequently used by GPs as an aid to the diagnosis of depression in the general population in primary care settings. It has also been adopted as one of the outcome measures for the evaluation of psychological treatment work within the Improved Access to Psychological Treatment (IAPT) programme in NHS adult mental health services in the UK. The PHQ-9 assesses both symptoms and current functioning. It is also easy to administer over the phone.

The PHQ-9 is recommended by:

■ *Understanding Mothers' Mental Health & Well-being During their Transition to Motherhood* (IHV, 2014).

■ NICE (2014) recommends that healthcare professionals in universal services should assess the level of contact and support needed by women with a mental health problem and those at risk of developing one (as identified at an initial assessment). For women who have been unwell before, and those who are receiving ongoing treatment (medical or psychological) they suggest that professionals discuss with a woman how her symptoms will be monitored and that the PHQ-9 is one of the self-report tools that might be used to do this.

Case example: Christina

Christina's son was born as a result of an unplanned pregnancy with her new partner. She had been working in a solicitor's office and was disappointed to have to give up work after her maternity leave because of childcare costs. Her energy levels became very low, she was worried about her teenage daughter and she found it increasingly difficult to go out, feeling that other mothers in her local area were judging her. It was harder still when her partner started working away from home and she missed his practical support at bath and bed time. Her GP suggested referral to a local family support project and prescribed antidepressants. At first Christina declined a visit from Family Action but when the antidepressants helped improve her motivation she agreed to accept their help.

4. The Community Practitioners and Health Visitors Association (CPHVA) 'How are you feeling?' booklets

This is an important resource for the assessment of the large number of new mothers in the UK who are from ethnic minorities, have motherhood practices that are divergent from British practices and who have little or no English. The booklets are a picture-based tool developed by Abi Sobowale, a senior health visitor, together with local communities in Sheffield. Health visitors in Sheffield were very aware that many ethnic groups expressed the concepts of depression and emotional well-being differently from the Western medical understanding which underpins tools like the EPDS. Developing this picture booklet tool in consultation with local women was a major undertaking and an exemplary bottom-up service development. Local non-English speaking women were involved in all stages of the project from conceptualisation to piloting and evaluation. Careful and respectful work involved the commissioned artist developing illustrations via community visits to clinical settings and women's homes.

The booklets were developed in Urdu, Bengali, Chinese, Somali and Arabic. Each booklet was deliberately compiled with simple engaging illustrations and non-'wordy' captions. There are pages depicting aches and pains, feelings of being low or wanting to hide away and being able or unable to enjoy food or company, for example (see Figure 3.1). Sobowale (2003) suggests that the booklets can be used at any stage in pregnancy and following childbirth. It is important to recognise that the booklets do not replace the need for interpreters or link workers. Where same-language link workers or community staff are looking at the booklets with a woman to explore how they are feeling, it is important that they report back to the professional who has responsibility for the care of the mother and her baby.

The 'How are you feeling?' booklets are recommended in the *Maternal Mental Health Pathway* (Department of Health, 2012). This guidance recommends ensuring good communication by being aware of cultural sensitivities to mental health and the use of appropriately trained interpreters and written materials designed for the purpose such as the picture booklets. See an example page from the Arabic booklet in Figure 3.1 below.

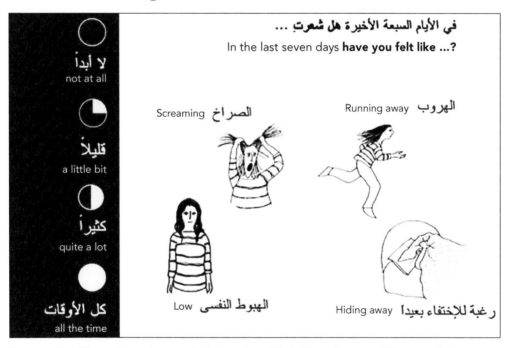

Figure 3.1: Page from CPHVA Arabic booklet. Reprinted with permission from Sobowale A (2003) *Perinatal Mental Health – New Resources for Supporting Non-English Speaking Women*. Community Practitioners and Health Visitors Association (CPHVA) Conference proceedings, October 2003.

It is important that professionals extend their knowledge of other cultures as much as possible, either through formal training or sharing across teams or local groups and ethnic minority organisations. Many of these groups have mental health promotion workers or offer counselling. Sobowale compiled a useful list of key points to remember when working with non-English speaking women.

'*Key points to remember when working with non-English speaking women.*

■ *Expressing cultural and religious identity is a basic human right.*

■ *Being a member of a minority cultural group can have a significant impact on your mental health. Be aware of the impact of racism on the lives of ethnic minority people.*

■ *Everyone belongs to a culture, within every culture there are sub-cultures.*

■ *Try to understand other people's cultures and be aware of your own cultural assumptions and how they may affect your response to people of a different culture.*

■ *Make sure you know how mental illness is regarded in that culture, sufferers are often stigmatised. Discuss mood not depression.*

■ *Treat people as individuals, avoid stereotyping and/or generalisation and find out their preferences.*

■ *Religious beliefs and practices are central to the lives of many ethnic minority people in Britain, even those born and brought up in Britain.*

■ *Family may be organised and shaped by cultural and religious tradition.*

■ *There are gender role differences, women usually look after the family.*

■ *Language and communication are two key barriers to equality of access to health services by ethnic minority people.*

■ *Work in partnership with black and ethnic minority communities and organisations.*

■ *Psychological distress may go unrecognised because of different ways of conceptualising illness, health and mental health.*

■ *Childbearing is important and elevates a woman's status.*

■ *Gender of the baby is important and may be a very sensitive issue in the family, males usually being favoured.*

■ *Be open and honest and try to give information in the language of choice.*

■ *The same stressful life events occur in every culture but different cultures have developed different ways of dealing with them.*'

(Reprinted with permission from Sobowale A (2003) *Perinatal Mental Health – New Resources for Supporting Non-English Speaking Women.* Community Practitioners and Health Visitors Association (CPHVA) Conference proceedings, October 2003.)

5. The antenatal and postnatal promotional guides

The promotional guide system was developed from the European Early Promotional Project (EEPP) which had developed a new partnership approach for health visitors and family nurses working with parents and families. The style of professional approach that the guides promote is a partnership with parents, with providers aiming to use:

- attentive listening

- matched agendas

- open, exploratory prompts

- shared decisions, goals and actions

- open agreements and disagreements

- a balance of guiding, leading and following

- avoiding a shift to expert judgement.

(Davis *et al*, 2010)

The antenatal promotional guide helps parents think about their own experiences of being brought up, their expectations for their children and any positive changes they might want to make to improve their own health and well-being. The postnatal promotional guide can help health visitors work with parents to promote secure attachment between parents and their newborns and to identify emotional issues that might need early support. It also encourages parents to use reflective functioning (see also Chapter 6), such as encouraging parents to wonder 'What do you think your baby might be feeling?'

The promotional guide system is used extensively by health visitors in England who have been trained in the approach. The guides are a structured, manualised approach for practitioners to work on the transition of mothers and fathers to parenthood, the early development of babies and the assessment of need and joint planning for professionals and families.

Case example: Monica

Monica was sexually abused by her father as a child. She never disclosed this and because she tried to run away from home she was labelled by her family as 'difficult'. In her 30s she was happy to meet and marry a man with whom she had a baby. She had been troubled by obsessive cleaning before she married but after the baby was born it became much more severe. She spent a great deal of time cleaning the flat and could not leave home without showering and washing her hair. She felt sad how little time she was making to play with her daughter. For her baby's sake she attended the local children's centre. She felt unable to chat to other mothers because she felt they were only interested in gossip. A family support worker noticed how tense she looked and made her a cup of coffee and asked if there was anything she was worried about. Because she knew she needed help, Monica was able to tell her she was worried about her excessive cleaning and they were able to arrange a referral to local psychology services.

The Wellbeing Plan

This is a new tool developed by Boots Family Trust Alliance (2013b) whose partners include the Royal College of Midwives and the Institute of Health Visiting. It is designed to extend the idea of birth planning, which focuses on labour and delivery, to emotional health and well-being and intends to help put mental and physical health on an equal footing. It was developed in response to the Boots Family Trust's survey findings that midwives and health visitors wanted more written materials to facilitate discussion and treatment of maternal mental health difficulties.

The tool highlights for women that they may be having mixed emotions about pregnancy and their baby. It suggests that some common signs that they should talk through with their midwife or health visitor are:

- tearfulness
- feeling overwhelmed
- being irritable/arguing more often
- lack of concentration
- change in appetite
- problems sleeping or extreme energy
- racing thoughts

- feeling more anxious

- lack of interest in usual things.

It suggests women think about the sorts of approaches to help them cope that might appeal to them most, such as:

- Talking to someone they trust about how they feel, such as a parent, sibling, partner or trusted friend.

- Asking for help with things at home, like chores and babysitting.

- Discussing the possibility of counselling or medication with their GP.

The Wellbeing Plan asks parents-to-be and new parents to think about their strengths and vulnerabilities and who in their family and network might be in a position to offer help and support. It is a practical, user-friendly tool which both increases awareness of mental health issues during pregnancy and after birth, and acts as a good prompt for women and their partners to have conversations about these areas. Like the traditional birth plan, the Wellbeing Plan has space for women and their partners to record their particular fears and worries and write down sources of support and help that would be most acceptable to them.

The Boots Family Trust Alliance (2013b) recommend that The Wellbeing Plan should be made available to all women during the third trimester. This is most likely to be done by a woman's midwife. They emphasise that focusing on mental well-being in pregnancy should be as routine as discussions of physical health.

A suggested interview structure for Postnatal Mental Health Assessment

This interview structure was developed by the author in collaboration with a tri-lingual health visitor (who spoke English, Arabic and Amharic (spoken in Ethiopia)), as part of a service development project in Camden, London. The project aimed to better address the needs assessment of Arabic speaking women and mothers in the borough. If a midwife, health visitor, community nursery nurse or link worker share a common language with a non-English speaking mother or are able to talk to a mother at some length with an interpreter, this is a very useful structure to follow to make a fairly comprehensive mental health assessment.

Maternal mental health assessments – suggested interview structure

The interview should ideally look at both the mental functioning (i.e. mental health or otherwise) and the day-to-day functioning (i.e. how time is spent, management of the tasks of daily living) as good information in both these areas gives a comprehensive mental health assessment.

If any clues about previous mental health history emerge, then information on previous difficulties (i.e. diagnosis/nature and extent of difficulties) and any treatment offered (e.g. medication, hospital admission, therapy/counselling) is relevant to the assessment of how the woman is presenting now.

1. Mental functioning

Ask about feelings, thoughts and behaviour (i.e. what she is actually doing).

- Feelings – look for feelings such as numb, low, not caring, lack of interest, hopeless, anxious, fearful, irritable.

- Thoughts – look for ideas of guilt, low self-worth, bleak outlook, self-blaming, statements about hopelessness. Pre-occupations/exaggerated worries about own health, baby's health, baby's vulnerability.

- Behaviour – look for anxious over-activity, inability to motivate herself to do basic tasks, letting other people take over, inability to decide what to do, preoccupation with one activity over any other.

2. Day-to-day functioning

- Looking after self (sleep, eating, hygiene, exercise, doing something she enjoys).

- Looking after baby (what is she doing and how is it going?).

- Social contact (who does she spend time with, who is she able to talk to/ confide in?).

3. Adjustment

Adjusting to a new baby (first or subsequent children) is a challenge to emotional health for all mothers. How is this mother managing?

- New family relationships.

- Lack of outside work routine or her previous life outside the home.

- Less time for self.

- Give and take with partner and sharing of tasks.

- New role and self-image.

- Changing ideas about what is important.

- Other losses, e.g. financial, appearance.

Obviously an interview with a new mother, especially if there are language difficulties or it is conducted through an interpreter, will not be able to cover all these areas – this is just a guide. However, asking open questions in these sorts of areas and following up what a woman says spontaneously on these topics will go a long way towards getting a picture of whether she may be showing symptoms of postnatal depression.
(Gellhorn, 2002, unpublished)

Overview of good practice for maternal mental health assessment

Taking note of information from other sources

It is important to always remember that no assessment tool is an assessment in itself. Assessment needs to be an ongoing process, especially as new mothers progress on their motherhood journey. It is important to take note of information from other sources. These might include observations at a baby clinic, frequency of GP and paediatric consultations, police reports regarding domestic disturbance or assaults and information about housing or difficulties at nursery.

Women's reported experience of detection and assessment

In a 2013 survey of 1,500 women, almost a third reported that they had never told a health professional that they felt unwell (Boots Family Trust, 2013a). Because perinatal mental health difficulties can present with a wide range of symptoms, women can struggle to understand what is wrong. In the same survey, professionals agreed that women's partners are likely to pick up the signs of mental health problems before the woman herself is able to recognise that things are not as normal. In an Australian study (Small *et al*, 1994) researchers demonstrated women's positive and negative experiences of seeking professional help. Women with positive experiences appreciated health professionals who gave them time, acknowledged their feelings and offered support.

'Not that she [the health professional] offered any miraculous cure, but I felt she really understood what I was talking about. That was helpful.'

'Once I'd spoken to them [doctor and maternal and child health nurse] I think I felt much better, you know, once I'd spoken and admitted that I wasn't coping really well, I felt so much better.'
(Small *et al*, 1994)

In contrast, other women showed that when their feelings were denied and when they felt unable or were not given the opportunity to talk, the experience of seeking help can be very negative.

Checklist for maternal mental health assessments

1. Ensure access to a quiet, private, appropriate space to conduct the assessment conversation.

2. Establish optimum trust and rapport with a woman before the assessment. Ideally this will be a mother with whom you have had previous contact as this will increase the likelihood that she will share information about her mental well-being with you.

3. Introduce the assessment tool and rationale for its use, if you are using one.

4. Ask the woman if she is agreeable to complete the tool with you.

5. Take account of and respect individual circumstances and cultural practices.

6. Assess any risk of harm to mother and baby (follow any local safeguarding procedures as appropriate).

7. Make clinical judgements about very low scores or extreme high scores (e.g. a woman scoring zero on the EPDS is likely to be disguising how she is really feeling).

8. Communicate your assessment sensitively to the woman and share with partner and family members if appropriate.

9. Plan your communication with other professionals and services e.g. GP, perinatal mental health services. Always think about what follow up you and others will need to offer if mental health needs are revealed.

10. Initiate a discussion with the woman about treatment options and the availability of sources of additional support locally.

Dealing with suicidal ideation

Asking questions about self-harm is not easy. The EPDS is helpful in this respect because item 10 puts a question about self-harm in black and white.

'*10. The thought of harming myself has occurred to me:*
- *Yes, quite often.*
- *Sometimes.*
- *Hardly ever.*
- *Never.*'
(The EPDS Scale, Cox *et al*,1987)

Even if a woman is not feeling suicidal, prompting a discussion about times when she feels at the end of her tether is helpful. Any positive response to item 10 in the EPDS requires further attention to the thoughts and feelings behind the woman's response and action to safeguard her from risk to herself, if needed. Assessing suicidality is a skilled task in mental health but important initial enquiries can seek to evaluate the following areas.

Previous history

Has she made any previous suicide attempts? Is there any family history of suicide? Both these factors increase the current risk of suicide.

Suicide plans

Having an actual plan of how to commit suicide (e.g. 'I would take all the tablets in my bathroom cabinet') indicates greater risk than just a report that someone has had thoughts of suicide (e.g. 'I sometimes feel I want to end it all').

Means and access

A woman's access to the means to commit suicide can vary significantly. For example a pharmacist or doctor will have access to dangerous drugs, a woman may live near to a high speed railway line. Family members may be able to limit access to the means to commit suicide in the short term while psychiatric assessment or inpatient care is arranged.

The CMACE report (Oates & Cantwell, 2011) warns against equating suicide risk with socio-economic deprivation. In their report over half the maternal suicide cases were women who were white, married, employed, living in comfortable circumstances and aged 30 years or over (see also Chapter 9)

Presence of the following factors increases the risk of suicide (see also Chapter 8).

■ The presence of severe mental illness (e.g. postpartum psychosis, bipolar disorder).

■ The presence of personality disorder and/or history of impulsive behaviour.

■ Alcohol or substance abuse.

■ The presence of domestic violence.

Protective factors include:

■ good family support

■ a woman being agreeable to a shared treatment plan or care plan

■ a woman being accepting of increased social support.

It is important for all workers to be aware that talking to a woman about suicidal ideation is not going to make her more likely to harm herself.

Evidence of suicidal thoughts? Inform and refer to the woman's GP for further evaluation.

Concern about immediate suicide risk? Arrange for supervision of the woman and her baby until an urgent psychiatric assessment can be arranged via an accident and emergency department or local perinatal psychiatry team if there is one in your area.

Managing tears

In Western culture there is significant pressure not to express feelings through tears in public and sometimes, especially for men, even in private. This is in contrast to other parts of the world, where public wailing and tearing at one's clothing would be an expected response to loss and grief. This cultural pressure of the 'stiff upper lip' approach to adversity and emotional pain can contribute to mental health difficulties at a later date. For example suppression of grief can lead to panic attacks arising some months on for someone who has tried too hard to 'be strong'.

Being able to cry, especially alongside someone who does not deny or try to minimise the pain, can validate a woman's experience and give her a sense of value. A health professional's acceptance of her current feelings of unhappiness may give her an opportunity to face her difficulties. This in turn may enable her to move forward to a different stage of thinking and coping. In these moments it is most helpful if caregivers are able to resist the urge to:

- comfort (e.g. saying 'I know you feel awful today, but look at how beautiful your baby is.')

- reassure (e.g. 'You feel awful now but you will recover from this soon enough.')

- offer advice ('It's sunny today, perhaps you could take the baby out this afternoon.').

It is important to note that many women will be tearful at various points in pregnancy and new motherhood without being depressed or otherwise suffering from mental health difficulties. Reviewing your assessment over time will differentiate transient distress from emotional health difficulties which need more attention (see Chapter 5).

Conclusion

The starting point for all health professionals should be the facilitation of women talking about their experience and the professional being prepared to take the time to hear her story.

- Taking the opportunity – the many health contacts and non-statutory services offered to women in pregnancy and when they have a newborn offer a window of opportunity for assessment of emotional well-being. Many women may have had pre-existing difficulties and will be particularly open to accepting help with these when they are motivated to do their best for their baby.

- Taking the time – many findings show that what is valued by women is professionals taking the time to talk to them and hear about their experiences and feelings. This is the best basis for good detection of maternal mental health difficulties.

- Use recommended assessment tools – national and professional guidelines recommend their use as part of a clinical assessment. Many women have mental health difficulties which can be missed or misdiagnosed which means that these women and their babies are not offered the treatment and additional support which they may need (Jones & Shakespeare, 2014).

- If properly introduced and sensitively administered most women find these tools acceptable. Many services currently use the Whooley questions as an initial assessment or screen for risk followed up with the EPDS or HADS as part of a fuller clinical assessment if mental health difficulties are identified.

- If your local area does not have a clear policy or pathway for maternal mental health difficulties and their detection, form a multi-agency working group to develop one.

■ With due regard to appropriate confidentiality, communicate with other professionals or community workers who may have contact with the woman you are seeing. They may have information about how she is doing in another setting.

■ Maternal mental health assessment is not a one off task – all contacts should be used to review emotional health and well-being of mother and baby. Many women may experience new difficulties in late pregnancy or well into their first year of motherhood. Midwives, GPs and health visitors should always share information about mental health history and emerging concerns so that a full picture of a woman's actual difficulties can be gained.

References

Beck AT, Ward CH, Mendelson M, Mock J & Erbaugh J (1961) An inventory for measuring depression. *Archives of General Psychiatry* **4** 561–571.

Boots Family Trust Alliance (2013a) *Perinatal Mental Health: Experiences of women and health professionals* [online]. Available at: http://www.bftalliance.co.uk/the-report/ (accessed April 2016).

Boots Family Trust Alliance (2013b) *My Pregnancy and Post-birth Well-being Plan* [online]. Available at: http://everyonesbusiness.org.uk/wp-content/uploads/2014/06/Boots-Family-Trust-Well-being-Plan. pdf (accessed April 2016).

Cox JL, Holden JM & Sagovsky R (1987) Detection of postnatal depression. Development of the 10-item Edinburgh Postnatal Depression Scale. *British Journal of Psychiatry* **150** (6) 782–786.

Coyle B & Adams C (2002) The EPDS: guidelines for its use as part of a maternal mental health assessment. *Community Practitioner* **75** (10) 394–395.

Davis H, Dusoir T, Papadopoulou P, Dimitrakaki C, Cox C, Ispanovic-Radojkovic V, Puura K, Vizacou S, Paradisiotou A, Rudic N, Chisholm B, Leontiou F, Mäntymaa M, Radosavljev J, Davis H & Day C (2010) *Working in Partnership with Parents* (2nd edition). London: Pearson.

Department of Health (2012) *Maternal Mental Health Pathway* (Best Practice Guidance) [online]. Available at: https://www.gov.uk/government/uploads/system/uploads/attachment_data/file/212906/ Maternal-mental-health-pathway-090812.pdf (accessed April 2016).

Gellhorn S (2002) Unpublished manuscript. Structured Interview for Maternal Mental Health Assessment.

Hill C (2010) *An Evaluation of Screening for Postnatal Depression Against NSC Criteria*. National Screening Committee. Available at: http://legacy.screening.nhs.uk/postnataldepression (accessed April 2016).

Howard LM, Molyneaux E, Dennis C-L, Rochat T, Stein A & Milgrom J (2014) Non-psychotic disorders in the perinatal period. *Lancet* **384** (9956) 1775–1788.

Institute of Health Visiting (2014) *Understanding Mothers' Mental Health & Well-Being During Their Transition To Motherhood. Good Practice Points for Health Visitors* [online]. Available at: http://ihv.org. uk/wp-content/uploads/2015/09/GPP_Mothers-Mental-health_V4-WEB.pdf (accessed April 2016)

Institute for Health Visiting (2015) *A National Framework For Continuing Professional Development For Health Visitors* [online]. Available at: http://ihv.org.uk/wp-content/uploads/2015/09/iHV_ Framework-CPD-standardsAW-WEB.pdf (accessed April 2016)

Jones I & Shakespeare J (2014) Easily missed? Postnatal depression. *BMJ* **349** g4500.

Mann R, Adamson J & Gilbody SM (2012) Diagnostic accuracy and case-finding questions to identify perinatal depression. *CMAJ* **184** (8) E424–E430.

Maternal Mental Health Alliance (2013) *Specialist Mental Health Midwives: What they do and why they matter* [online]. Available at: http://www.baspcan.org.uk/files/MMHA%20SMHMs%20Report.pdf (accessed April 2016).

Milgrom J, Mendelsohn J & Gemmill AW (2011) Does postnatal depression screening work? Throwing out the bathwater, keeping the baby. *Journal of Affective Disorders* **132** (3) 301–310.

Morrell CJ, Warner R, Slade P, Dixon S, Walters S, Paley G, Brugha T (2009) Psychological interventions for postnatal depression: cluster randomised trial and economic evaluation. The PoNDER trial. *Health Technology and Assessment* **13** (3) 1–153.

NICE (2014) *Antenatal and Postnatal Mental Health: Clinical management and service guidance* [online]. Available at: https://www.nice.org.uk/guidance/cg192 (accessed April 2016).

Oates M & Cantwell R (2011) Deaths from psychiatric causes. In: Centre for Maternal and Child Enquiries (CMACE) Saving Mothers' Lives: Reviewing Maternal Deaths To Make Motherhood Safer: 2006-08. *BJOG* **118** (S1) 1–203.

Shakespeare J, Blake F & Garcia J (2003) A qualitative study of the acceptability of routine screening of postnatal women using the Edinburgh Postnatal Depression Scale. *British Journal of General Practice* **53** (493) 614–619.

Small R, Brown S & Lumley J (1994) Missing voices: what women say and do about depression after childbirth. *Journal of Reproductive and Infant Psychology* **12** 89–103.

Sobowale A (2003) *Perinatal Mental Health – New Resources for Supporting Non-English Speaking Women*. Community Practitioners and Health Visitors Association (CPHVA) conference proceedings, October 2003.

Whooley MA, Avins AL, Miranda J & Browner WS (1997) Case-finding instruments for depression. Two questions are as good as many. *Journal of General Internal Medicine* **12** (7) 439–445. Available at: http://www.ncbi.nlm.nih.gov/pmc/articles/PMC1497134/ (accessed April 2016).

Zigmond AS & Snaith RP (1983) The hospital anxiety and depression scale. *Acta Psychiatrica Scandinavica* **67** (6) 361–370.

Chapter 4: Levels of intervention, treatment and support

Sue Gellhorn

Introduction

Recent reports of the costs of perinatal mental health problems indicate that in the UK we are a long way off providing adequate care and services for women with perinatal mental health difficulties (Bauer *et al*, 2014). This is particularly the case for the more specialist services, such as perinatal mental health teams and mother and baby units. However, the quantity and quality of provision at the level of universal services also varies and depends on the case load pressures and vacancy rates for key posts. It also depends on the local management and policy commitment to the needs of women with these sorts of difficulties.

This chapter will introduce a range of interventions and ways of supporting women with perinatal mental health difficulties. These will be broadly arranged in terms of the level or 'intensity' of the support or intervention, from self-help and self-care to intensive home visiting and community treatment approaches. While talking to and supporting women and their babies, the importance of a multi-pronged or mixed 'package' approach should be kept in mind. We are used to a world of treatment standards, best practice guidelines and evidence-based practice. However, more than in any other area of community health, in maternal mental health care, one approach really doesn't suit all.

For example, women may say:

'I don't want counselling but I would like help to get out of the house more than I do.'
Or:
'I'm no good in groups but I would like to go somewhere where my baby can play with other children and socialise.'

Levels of intervention

Mental health prevention and promotion

When understanding and knowledge of maternal mental health (and the risk factors for postnatal depression in particular) was extending in the 1990s, it stimulated an interest in preventative interventions which might be offered antenatally to mothers considered to be at risk. However, translating risk factor research into preventive strategies is not straightforward because complex interactions of risk factors and individual variations are involved. There have been numerous studies exploring preventative interventions, which have had mixed results. However a recent Cochrane review of a very large number of studies (Dennis & Dowswell, 2013) concluded that there was evidence that a number of approaches were helpful for prevention. These were:

- professionally-based home visiting (such as intensive nursing home visits)
- flexible postnatal care by midwives
- postnatal peer-based telephone support
- interpersonal psychotherapy.

Dennis and Dowswell noted that both the midwifery-led postnatal care and the peer telephone support studies incorporated screening with the Edinburgh Postnatal Depression Scale (EPDS) for the early identification of depressive symptoms. They note that interventions targeting 'at risk' mothers are more likely to be feasible than those offered generically. They also made a recommendation that interventions target migrant women because they appear to be at greater risk of developing depression, and also women's partners, because of the impact of partner support on depression in mothers.

However extensive or limited prevention approaches are, women's reported experience of postnatal depression and other mental health difficulties is that they would have felt better prepared, less frightened and more able to seek support and help if they had been better informed about perinatal mental health difficulties.

Psychoeducation

Psychoeducation is an important element of many psychosocial interventions for maternal mental health difficulties. Giving information about a mental health condition and how it may present is especially helpful for early self-identification. As noted in Chapter 3, women often feel that things are not right but are unsure as to the nature of their difficulties. In addition, information about social support and treatments available (community-based and more medical) can remove a simple barrier to women accessing help, i.e. knowing what is available in their local area and how to go about accessing it.

Psychoeducation can also help through normalisation of women's experience. With good information about emotional well-being and pregnancy and motherhood, women are able to recognise that they are not 'going mad' or a bad mother but may be experiencing mental health difficulties common to a significant group of women (perinatal depression 7-14%, perinatal anxiety 8-15%) (Heron *et al*, 2004). The information provided online and as downloadable leaflets by the Royal College of Psychiatrists and by Mind are excellent examples.

Self-care

Struggling to care for oneself in addition to a baby is often a factor in the development of maternal mental health difficulties. Giving support so that a woman can meet her own needs is a very valuable intervention. Or even pointing out to her that it is perfectly valid for her to meet her own needs as well as her baby's. Encouraging her to accept offers of babysitting from relatives, friends or neighbours can give a new mother a short break to visit the hairdresser or see a friend which can lift her mood. In exceptional circumstances, where such social support is not available, arranging a part time emergency child minding or nursery place can provide relief. However this needs to be carefully balanced with the need to support a vulnerable mother's attachment to her newborn. The significance of self-care reflects an important understanding that underpins many key findings in the literature on mothering and women's mental health. This is that, where women are well taken care of themselves (however they are supported), the care, particularly emotional care, that they are able to offer their babies is maximised.

The Mind website offers a helpful list of suggestions to women under the heading 'What can I do to help myself?' (Mind, 2014)

These include:

- *'Getting adequate rest and sleep.*
- *Eating well.*
- *Taking regular exercise.*
- *Taking time out for oneself e.g. reading a magazine, having a relaxing bath.*

■ *Keeping in touch with social support e.g. talking to close friends, socialising with other mothers, confiding in someone about how you are feeling.'*

(Mind, 2014)

Listening visits

Listening visits were developed as a first level talking treatment delivered by health visitors and other community health staff in the 1980s and 1990s. This work was linked to policies aiming to improve the detection of maternal mental health difficulties, focusing on depression in the postnatal period. Where this was well developed and successful, there were clear decision steps and pathways for care. In the best service models, health staff had regular clinical supervision with a mental health expert and there was good management support for the work.

Listening visits are a natural extension of the importance of giving women time to talk about how they are feeling and gain their trust, a factor that has been mentioned time and again in reports about obstacles to good professional support for women in difficulty (Hogg, 2013; Department of Health, 2013).

A third year student midwife reports:

'Women appear not to declare their low mood, I think this is because we rush through questions and don't create an environment for discussion because we don't have the time. The only woman who has shared mental health worries was one I gave an hour to. It took that long to earn her trust.'
(Royal College of Midwives, 2014)

Listening visits are a dedicated time to visit a new mother and listen to how she is getting on in her new role, the difficulties she is experiencing, how she is feeling about herself, her new identity as a mother and her relationship with her new baby. The focus of the meeting is not to find solutions or take action, but to hear about her experience and validate her feelings. The skills required are those needed to be with someone in distress without rushing to fix or reassure, which can be difficult if your training is within medical approaches and you have a strong professional instinct to 'make things better'. Similarly, women will report the helpfulness of a GP who will take time to listen rather than feel a pressure to 'help' by reaching for the prescription pad.

The task is the 'containment' of the woman's feelings (and your own) as you listen to her story. Containment describes the work through which practitioners are encouraged to help process emotions and anxieties that are felt to be overwhelming for their clients and will be considered again in Chapter 6. This very much represents a mirroring of the emotional task of a new mother who has the job of attending to her baby's distress, doing her best to understand his upset and helping the baby to feel that his feelings are manageable and not overwhelming. A big part of parenting is helping a child see the world and his experiences in it as a stimulating but manageable place. In the very beginning, as a newborn, the baby's feelings are very primitive and powerful. Similarly, the emotional terrain for a new parent can feel rocky and unexpectedly powerful. It is providing a listening ear to this powerful, and at times overwhelming, experience that can help a new mother feel held and supported so that she can feel able to manage her baby's emotional life alongside her own new emotional learning curve.

'If someone had told me that a professional could come every week and let me talk for half an hour, and that I would end up a healed person, I wouldn't have believed it. It sounds nonsense, but it's true.'
(A mother's experience of home-based listening support from a trained health visitor, Holden *et al*, 1989)

Community support as treatment

Some of the services, peer support initiatives and 'empowerment' opportunities offered through Sure Start, and now in children's centres, build a great deal on the understanding and community psychology approaches pioneered by psychotherapist Sue Holland in a deprived housing estate in White City, west London in the late 1980s. In a community psychology approach the empowering of communities is seen as the key to both ameliorating and preventing mental distress. This is in contrast to a traditional medical approach which offers clinical solutions to disorders in individuals. The White City project saw the task as moving women from receiving therapeutic help and support to taking action in their own local community by developing peer support. Sue Holland reminded professionals and sceptical colleagues in the psychotherapy world that depression literally means 'being put down, lowered'. Putting together her psychotherapy training and her very 'hands-on' involvement with the women she was helping, she saw that:

'...by way of this networking on the estate, each woman can discover that she is not uniquely mad, bad, or alone in her private symptoms, but shares common suffering and collective strengths with other women.'
(Holland, 1994)

This pioneering work paved the way for lots of excellent community services for women today. Some examples of work in children's centres using community support to improve maternal mental health are outlined below.

1. My Time My Space

Creativity Works is a voluntary sector arts organisation that works with partner organisations in health and children's centres in Somerset and the west of England to provide an art group called My Time My Space. The project is provided in a children's centre and facilitated by experienced artists supported by health visitors and children's centre staff. These groups exemplify a non-stigmatising therapeutic opportunity which prioritises giving mothers time and space to think about themselves and try something new. There is a crèche and mothers are able to relax, share with other mothers and focus on the art they are creating for a short while. Outcomes show improvements in mental well-being as measured by the Edinburgh Postnatal Depression Scale (Department of Health, 2015)

'There's a supportive artist who inspires you, there's a health visitor to support you and there are people who are similar to you to listen, to express. And there's time. But all of it added up together becomes more than that. A lot more than that.' (Participant in My Time My Space, www.creativity works.org.uk)

2. Raising Happy Babies

The adult psychology service offered within children's centres in Tower Hamlets, east London, worked hard to offer a more accessible service to new mothers and their families. They decided to offer a transition to parenthood course rather than a therapy group because there is evidence that this has been shown to increase access because it is perceived as less stigmatising and intimidating for participants, especially those from ethnic minorities where the stigma of mental health difficulties can be even greater. Through community consultation, a psychoeducation course for parents of babies from newborn to six months was named Raising Happy Babies (Marks *et al*, 2009).

A Sylheti-speaking assistant psychologist talked to local Bangladeshi women to find out what sort of name for the course would be most appealing to them. The course covers topics such as 'how babies communicate their feelings and needs', 'looking after yourself' and 'developing a support network'. The children's centres also do outreach work to explain the service to women and answer their questions to maximise attendance from women who are not accustomed to engaging in activities outside the home.

3. Strong Women

Children's centres in the north west of England offer group support for mothers with postnatal depression. The programme was developed through consultation with local health services, social care and local childcare providers. In Knutsford, Cheshire, they offer a six week 'Strong Women' programme which aims to build self-esteem, resilience and aspirations. Service users can go on to access a programme that has links with local industries and helps with further training and volunteering and work opportunities. Women who graduate from the programme are engaged in outreach work to help vulnerable women to access the 'Strong Women' courses and have a voice in the community to influence local policies (4Children, 2015).

Therapeutic services delivered by non-mental health specialists

A number of therapeutic intervention approaches make use of well-trained non-mental health staff working with individual women and families and with groups in children's centre settings and in the home. A number of approaches are introduced below and some will be considered in more detail in Chapter 6 and Chapter 12.

Mellow Babies

Mellow Parenting is a Scotland based charity who have developed parenting programmes which are based on attachment theory. One of the key elements of attachment theory is the concept of the transmission of attachment and relationship styles across generations. The Mellow Babies programme is an extension of this programme to offer an intervention for parents of under-ones who are felt to be vulnerable because of social and emotional needs, including anxiety and depression. Mellow Babies helps new mothers think about their own experience of being parented and how this has affected their own parenting style. The programme is also offered to some families where there are child protection concerns. Training is offered to health visitors and other community staff in delivering the programme.

Mellow Babies is a 14 week programme of one day attendance for mothers and babies to help them develop strong relationships with their new babies. The topics covered include:

- What do babies do all day?
- What can babies do?
- Bonding with baby.
- Emotional and social development.
- Sleep, playing, harmful parenting, safety in the home.

Fathers are invited to three evening sessions with content including psychoeducation about postnatal depression and activities to promote father-baby interaction. Mellow Babies aims to help parents deal with their own issues of poor relationships in their past and build positive interactions with their own babies through baby massage, singing songs and other interactive games (Puckering, 2009).

Family Nurse Partnership

The Family Nurse Partnership (FNP) is a home-based parenting programme that was adapted from a US programme originating from the University of Colorado. The American programme was very successful in improving outcomes for young single mothers living in socially deprived circumstances. FNP was brought to the UK following recommendations of the Social Exclusion Unit Task Force in 2006 and now provides services in 130 areas across the UK. FNP offers an intensive health visitor led programme targeted at low income, young, single, first time mothers (Rowe, 2009). Services are now commissioned by local authorities as part of their public health commitment for children aged 0-5 and are supported by the Family Nurse Partnership National Unit and Public Health England. Vulnerable new mothers are visited by a key worker through their pregnancy and up until their baby is two years old. The programme offers a combination of emotional and practical support in addition to education around child development and parenting. One of the key features of FNP that young mothers really value is the opportunity to build up a close and trusting relationship with their visiting family nurse so that they can be supported when things are difficult, but also their progress and successes can be celebrated with someone who knows them well.

The Solihull Approach

The Solihull Approach was developed in the 1990s by Hazel Douglas, a clinical psychologist and child psychotherapist working with a group of health visitors in Solihull on common infant difficulties with sleeping and eating. The Solihull Approach has now been applied to develop various parenting programmes across the UK (Douglas & Rheeston, 2009). Key health visiting staff are trained to engage with families in a partnership approach. The aim is to tackle early problems with sleeping, feeding and other difficulties with routine, before they lead on to future problems which might necessitate referral to child and adolescent mental health services (CAMHS). The three key concepts in the Solihull Approach are: containment, behaviour management and reciprocity. These concepts help the practitioners understand how a family's current situation is experienced by them and their baby before they offer intervention (see Chapter 12 for a fuller account). Parents are helped to have a better understanding of their baby's development and early communication so that ideas of reciprocity and waiting for your baby to be ready for more (food or interaction) facilitate positive attachment.

Family Action

Family Action is a voluntary sector organisation whose Perinatal Support Project (PSP) (Barlow & Coe, 2012) evolved out of the early work of Newpin (see Chapter 2). The work has been developed in four diverse pilot sites across the UK and aims to offer women experiencing perinatal anxiety and depression support from volunteer befrienders who have experienced perinatal mental health problems themselves. The PSP helps a group of women with a high level of need – a high proportion of single parent families, in no-wage households and with 2-11% having child protection issues. The project has successfully impacted on levels of anxiety and depression, social support and self-esteem.

Therapeutic services delivered by mental health specialists

Group therapy

Formal group therapy for postnatal women is unusual. However there are many forms of group therapeutic support that women may find beneficial. This ranges from structured psychoeducation groups for first time mothers to a targeted therapeutic group run by a therapist or counsellor for women referred by their midwife, health visitor or GP (Parkinson, 2009). For women, having their experiences validated by others and learning that they are not alone in their struggles are probably the most valuable experiences in such a group.

Couples therapy

It is likely that couples therapy is currently underused as an intervention for maternal mental health difficulties. Meeting a mother in difficulties with her partner can offer opportunities for psychoeducation, working on their communication and understanding their different childhood histories and how these have shaped their feelings about parenthood and their new baby. Communication and turn-taking listening strategies can be very useful tools for couples somewhat derailed by the intensity of feelings and challenges a newborn brings to their relationship.

Psychodynamic psychotherapy

Psychodynamic psychotherapy is unlikely to begin for a woman in the perinatal period unless it is offered within a specialist maternal mental health service where it may also involve sessions with her baby (see parent-infant psychotherapy). This therapy explores early childhood experiences and how they have shaped a woman's view of herself and her experience in relationships. It can be very helpful in helping a new mother understand where she can come unstuck in her relationships and how this may impact on her parenting.

Cognitive behavioural therapy

Cognitive behavioural therapy (CBT) is often seen as the treatment of choice for anxiety disorders, such as panic disorder, agoraphobia, social anxiety and obsessive compulsive disorder (NICE, 2014). CBT is widely available within NHS Improved Access to Psychological Therapy (IAPT) services. It is based on the idea that learned anxiety responses, thought patterns involving negative views of the self and negative predictions about future anxiety responses become an established pattern. CBT approaches can also be used for depression, where negative self-statements are challenged, and goals and homework are set in collaboration with the therapist to restore enjoyable activities and gradually improve mood. NICE recommend a stepped care approach to offering these treatments so that women with mild to moderate symptoms may be offered treatment via guided self-help in the first instance.

Interpersonal psychotherapy

Interpersonal psychotherapy (IPT) is a short-term therapy structured around understanding how low mood can arise as a result of difficulties in interpersonal functioning. One of four problem areas is chosen as a focus for the therapeutic work. These are: role transitions, role disputes, interpersonal sensitivity and grief. Many of these areas are very relevant problem areas for pregnant women and new mothers and IPT has been evaluated as an effective psychological treatment for perinatal depression and as such is also recommended in the antenatal and postnatal mental health guideline (NICE, 2014).

Compassionate mind therapy

Compassionate mind therapy approaches are relatively new but have a lot to offer women feeling low and judging themselves harshly in the perinatal period. Compassionate mind therapy makes use of a focus on compassion as an antidote to the shame and self-criticism often present for people with mental health difficulties, especially people who might have had neglectful, abusive or emotionally insecure backgrounds. By working on developing a 'compassionate self' and understanding that our emotional inheritance has shaped our critical self, the person can move to an approach to life that is less guilt ridden and where emotional regulation is achieved in a less defensive fashion. This sort of approach can resonate well for women where shame and guilt at not being a happy and contented new mother are part of the problem.

Mindfulness-based cognitive behavioural therapy

Mindfulness-based cognitive therapy is another relatively new psychological treatment derived from CBT and mindfulness-based stress reduction. It is often used with people who have recurrent depression and helps them become aware of the body sensations, thoughts and feelings associated with their episodes of depression. It cultivates a mindful approach to life and its challenges and a compassionate outlook on one's own limitations. There is growing evidence that it can also impact on parents' sensitivity and responsiveness to their children (Bailie *et al*, 2012). There is also new interest in applying the approach to antenatal preparation and in Oxford, trained midwives have offered mindfulness-based parent preparation courses (Wariner *et al*, 2012). The Royal College of Midwives recommends encouraging a mindful approach in supporting anxious or depressed pregnant women, noting that it can be helpful in slowing the body and mind and increasing feelings of being in control (Underdown & Barlow, 2012).

Parent-infant psychotherapy

Parent-infant psychotherapy (PIP) is a psychoanalytically informed therapy that is offered to mother and babies whose relationship (attachment) is in difficulty. The therapist works on the mother's difficulties, the infant's difficulties and the difficulties in their relationship throughout the therapy. The focus of the work is the interaction between the parent and baby. PIP is offered at specialist parent-infant projects which are slowly extending across the country (Baradon *et al*, 2005).

Medication

Medication as a treatment for women struggling with anxiety or depression as they attempt to deal with all the challenges of mothering and the domestic domain often gets a bad press. This is immortalised in the Rolling Stones' song about Valium in the 1960s, entitled 'Mother's Little Helper'. The over-use of benzodiazepines at that time links to a very wide debate about the medicalisation of women's problems with which the author has a lot of sympathy. However medication can play a very important role, and is sometimes essential in treating maternal mental health difficulties (see Chapter 9) as long as it is not seen as an automatic first port of call. A full account of the appropriate drugs, guidelines and prescription recommendations is beyond the scope of this volume (see NICE, 2014, and Chapters 9 and 11). Nevertheless, women will often need to talk about their thoughts and feelings about medication in relation to side effects, the balance of risks and benefits and breastfeeding. Talking through their feelings and choices alongside consulting with an expert prescriber, such as a perinatal psychiatrist, will be very helpful for some women.

Conclusion

This chapter has outlined the many points in the maternity journey and levels of service delivery where women with maternal mental health difficulties may benefit from intervention from care professionals they come into contact with. Some universal pointers to getting this right are:

Key points

1. It is key to recognise that perinatal mental health disorders and even perinatal depression are very heterogeneous in how they present, their aetiology and their context. Not surprisingly, the most effective help and intervention will vary depending on the woman and her baby.

2. Early detection of depression and other difficulties facilitates early intervention and treatment and is more likely to result in a favourable outcome for the mother, her baby, partner and family.

3. A multi-pronged treatment approach for depression is the most effective. Mild and moderate depression are often successfully treated with a combination of non-pharmacological treatments, not just one.

4. Psychoeducation can be an important help even after maternal mental health difficulties have been detected. The aim of psychoeducation is to help women and their families understand their symptoms, learn about available treatments and reinforce effective coping strategies.

References

4Children (2015) *The Future of Children's Centres and Opportunities to Maximise Their Potential* [online]. Children's Centre Census: A national overview of children's centres in 2015. Available at: http://www.4children.org.uk/Files/28082f59-4cb8-4116-a476-a536009e5d05/Children_Centre_Census_2015.pdf (accessed April 2016).

Bailie C, Kuyken W & Sonnenberg S (2012) The experiences of parents in mindfulness-based cognitive therapy. *Clinical Child Psychology and Psychiatry* **17** (1) 103–119.

Baradon T, Broughton C & Iris G (2005) *The Practice of Psychoanalytic Parent-Infant Psychotherapy: Claiming the baby*. Hove: Routledge.

Barlow J & Coe C (2012) *Family Action Perinatal Support Project: Research findings report* [online]. Warwick Medical School. Available at: https://www.family-action.org.uk/content/uploads/2014/06/Perinatal-Support-Project-evaluation-2012-Professor-Jane-Barlow.pdf (accessed April 2016).

Bauer A, Parsonage M, Knapp M, Lemmi V & Adelaja B (2014) *The Cost of Perinatal Mental Health Problems* [online]. PSSRU/Centre for Mental Health. Available at: http://eprints.lse.ac.uk/59885/1/__lse.ac.uk_storage_LIBRARY_Secondary_libfile_shared_repository_Content_Bauer,%20M_Bauer_Costs_perinatal_%20mental_2014_Bauer_Costs_perinatal_mental_2014_author.pdf (accessed April 2016).

Dennis CL & Dowswell T (2013) *Psychosocial and Psychological Interventions for Preventing Postpartum Depression* [online]. Available at: http://onlinelibrary.wiley.com/doi/10.1002/14651858.CD001134.pub3/abstract (accessed April 2016).

Department of Health (2013) *Health Visiting: the voice of service users. Learning from service users' experiences to inform the development of UK health visiting practice and services* [online]. National Nursing Research Unit, King's College London. Available at: https://www.kcl.ac.uk/nursing/research/nnru/publications/Reports/Voice-of-service-user-report-July-2013-FINAL.pdf (accessed April 2016).

Department of Health (2015) *High Impact Area 2: Maternal (perinatal) mental health. Health visitor programme*. Available at: https://www.gov.uk/government/uploads/system/uploads/attachment_data/file/424444/High_Impact_Area_2_V3.pdf (accessed April 2016).

Douglas H & Rheeston M (2009) The Solihull Approach: an integrative model across agencies. In: Barlow J and Svanberg PO (Eds) *Keeping the Baby in Mind* (pp 29-38). London: Routledge.

Heron J, O'Connor TG, Evans J, Glover V & ALSPAC Study Team (2004) The course of anxiety and depression through pregnancy and the post-partum in a community sample. *Journal of Affective Disorders* **80** (1) 65–73.

Hogg S (2013) *Prevention in Mind. All Babies Count: Spotlight on perinatal mental health* [online]. NSPCC. Available at: http://everyonesbusiness.org.uk/wp-content/uploads/2014/06/NSPCC-Spotlight-report-on-Perinatal-Mental-Health.pdf (accessed April 2016)

Holden JM, Sagovsky R & Cox J (1989) Counselling in a general practice setting: controlled study of health visitor intervention in the treatment of post-natal depression. *British Medical Journal* **298** 223–226.

Holland S (1994) From social abuse to social action: a neighbourhood psychotherapy and social action project for women. In: J Ussher and P Nicholson (Eds) *Gender Issues in Clinical Psychology* (pp68–77). London: Routledge.

Marks L, Hadley S, Reay A, Gelman T & McKay A (2009) Working with parents from black and minority ethnic backgrounds in children's centres. In: J Barlow and PO Svanberg (Eds) *Keeping the Baby in Mind* (pp128–138). London: Routledge.

Mind (2014) *Understanding Postnatal Depression* [online]. Available at: http://www.mind.org.uk/media/46890/understanding_postnatal_depression_2013.pdf (accessed April 2016).

NICE (2014) *Antenatal and Postnatal Mental Health: Clinical Management and Service Guidance* [online]. Available at: https://www.nice.org.uk/guidance/cg192 (accessed April 2016).

Parkinson K (2009) Giving birth to hope: group work for women with postnatal depression. *Healthcare Counselling and Psychotherapy Journal* **9** (3) 25–29.

Puckering C (2009) Mellow Babies: Mellow Parenting with parents of infants. In: Barlow J and Svanberg PO (Eds) *Keeping the Baby in Mind* (pp 155–163) London: Routledge.

Rowe A (2009) Perinatal home visiting: implementing the nurse-family partnership in England. In: J Barlow and PO Svanberg (Eds) *Keeping the Baby in Mind* (pp128–138). London: Routledge.

Royal College of Midwives (2014) *Pressure Points: Maternal Mental Health. Improving Emotional Wellbeing in Postnatal Care* [online]. Available at: https://www.rcm.org.uk/sites/default/files/Pressure%20Points%20-%20Mental%20Health%20-%20Final_0.pdf (accessed April 2016).

Underdown A & Barlow J (2012) *Maternal Emotional Wellbeing and Infant Development: A good practice guide for midwives* [online]. Royal College of Midwives. Available at: https://www.rcm.org.uk/sites/default/files/Emotional%20Wellbeing_Guide_WEB.pdf (accessed April 2016).

Wariner S, Williams M, Bardacke N & Dymond M (2012) A mindfulness approach to antenatal preparation. *British Journal of Midwifery* **20** (3) 194–198.

Chapter 5: Normal anxieties in early motherhood and those needing professional attention

Sue Gellhorn

In a busy clinic or community setting it is difficult to know which small clinical observations or feelings that something is 'not quite right' need further attention, thinking about or discussion with a colleague or other professional. This chapter is intended to help with the questions – 'How troubled is this mother?' or 'How worried should I be about her and her baby?'

Common worries

Worries about whether the baby is normal

Many women are worried in the first few moments, days, weeks or months about whether their baby is normal. There can be a number of reasons and emotional states underlying these fears and as mentioned before, sensitive listening and thoughtful exploration of a woman's fears is the approach needed. This concern can be around small skin blemishes, the shape of the features (which may be expressed as concern about disabilities such as Down's syndrome) or gastro-intestinal functioning (he or she is 'sick all the time' or 'does too many or too few poos' or poos of the wrong consistency or colour), or even gestures, eye movements or breathing patterns. The anxiety about the baby can be a result of a number of 'depressive' or 'paranoid' anxieties. As with the baby's own powerful and primitive early feelings these fears are very real and powerful for the new mother.

The mother may feel 'bad' inside because of earlier depression, domestic violence or a childhood that involved little warmth and confidence building. Because of these 'bad feelings' she may conclude that the baby coming from inside her body cannot be healthy and normal.

She may feel she has not been attentive enough, has had an instrumental birth, did not take enough care of herself in pregnancy and therefore feel she will be punished by having a baby who has difficulties too.

Some mothers may need little more than the affirmation of your own observations about her baby and how she interacts with him or her while others may need and be interested to have an opportunity to explore their feelings of doubt and inadequacy in a therapeutic setting.

Worries about being able to feed her baby

Breastfeeding initiatives in UK hospitals and support from midwives, health visiting and breastfeeding support volunteers have done much to increase the number of mothers successfully feeding their newborns. However there are many worries that can emerge about the feeding relationship. For example: 'I don't have enough milk to satisfy my baby.'

This can be an expression of anxiety about meeting the sometimes overwhelming demands of a new baby. The breastfeeding mother can feel depleted and anxious about her newborn's dependency on her own body and the quality of her breast milk.

If a mother is having difficulties with breastfeeding it can be experienced as a deeply personal hurt. As Roszika Parker noted in her in-depth examination of 'maternal ambivalence': 'Mothers (can) feel dominated, exploited, humiliated, drained and criticised by their babies.' (Parker, 2005). Responding helpfully to all of this involves taking the time needed to hear her worry, feel something of its depth and not rush to reassure. It is helpful to explore with her what might have made her think this and who she has to help and support her in persevering with or adjusting her feeding approach or exploring her worries further. A supportive partner can help reassure the nursing mother in times of difficulty, but failing that a listening health worker can overcome this trouble spot too: 'If I said to her, "Oh, I gave her a bottle last night" she wouldn't judge me…' (service user experience, Department of Health, 2013).

Worries about getting it right all the time or being the perfect mother

This can be expressed as fears that the baby is not happy with something that she is doing or is not getting their needs met. For example 'He doesn't like being in his crib, he hates being bathed, I don't have an expensive mechanical rocker'. This sort of worry is often voiced by mothers with perfectionistic tendencies and mothers who have had more than the usual professional involvement, for example where a baby initially has jaundice, was premature or needed to be nursed in a special care baby unit.

Again, hearing how hard it is to suddenly only have your own judgements of what the baby needs or is feeling, without the back-up of expert opinion, is important.

Worries about harming their baby

A more extreme version of the anxieties of being perfect, but also sometimes a sign of a more specific maternal mental health difficulty, is a mother expressing that she is worried about causing harm to her baby. This worry may be an extreme form of the worry that things are not 'good enough' for the baby (its care, the quality of its sleep or the stimulation she provides). Mothers may worry that their angry thoughts and feelings are harmful to the baby. For example feeling furious with their baby's wakefulness in the middle of the night and having the impulse to shake him or put him back rather roughly in his cot.

This worry is a concern about managing the ambivalence of everyday motherhood. A mother may feel ok about being snappy and critical with her partner but distressed about having angry feelings towards her baby. Listening to this and helping a woman think through the coping strategies she is using, the self-care steps she can put in place, and the practical support and professional help she can call on will help her contain this anxiety.

However, if the hostility towards the baby seems to predominate and the mother's compassion for the baby seems lacking, then safeguarding concerns would need to be raised. This is especially important where there is minimal social support and other social adversity factors are present (see the 'toxic trio' in Chapter 8).

Ambivalent feelings that are very strongly resisted can emerge in the form of obsessional thoughts about harming her baby through an overly hot bath, smothering or with sharp objects. The more these intrusive images or thoughts occur the more anxious the woman may become. This level of difficulty is the presentation of postnatal obsessional compulsive disorder (OCD) and will be considered more fully in chapter 10. In this case a woman will need referral to a clinical psychologist for psychological treatment.

Worrying they are not 'in love' with their baby

The Royal College of Midwives (RCM) good practice guide on maternal emotional well-being (Underdown & Barlow, 2012) reports that as many women as one in five may experience difficulties bonding with their baby. This can be associated with very strong feelings of guilt, shame and inadequacy. Without understanding and sensitive handling this can build into something that affects all aspects of early care and colours the mother's experience of early motherhood.

Women expressing worries about this may be premature in their concern – noticing they have not felt the rush of powerful, unconditional love they had expected, read about or heard from other mothers' accounts or indeed experienced themselves with earlier births. They may be one of the many women who, being exhausted and sore after delivery, feel rather flat but grow to develop a close connection with their baby as the relationship develops. Others may be suffering from post-traumatic disorder (PTSD), may be numb with grief following a major bereavement or, later on in the baby's life, be bravely reporting that something does indeed feel missing in their relationship with this baby.

The RCM guide gives steps for midwives to take to promote early bonding post-delivery, for instance time to get to know each other before non-urgent medical procedures and skin-to-skin holding. Baby massage classes have helped many mothers improve their sense of close connectedness with their babies. More serious difficulties with bonding and attachment may require referral to a parent-infant psychotherapy resource (see PIP UK voluntary sector resources and NHS services such as the Perinatal and Parent Infant Mental Health services at Chelsea and Westminster Hospital (CNWL) and Goodmayes Hospital (NELFT)) which work specifically with difficulties in the mother-baby relationships.

Case example: Lorraine

Lorraine was a single mother of a two-year-old girl and a six-month-old boy. She was barely pregnant with her son when the father of both children died suddenly from an undiagnosed heart condition. There was lots of family upset and having been someone in the family who always supported others, she found it hard to express her grief and ask for help for herself. She wanted to support her toddler daughter with her loss and felt that the new baby was something she managed in a practical way but with little involvement. One day, feeling very tired and a little resentful, she handled him rather roughly and recognised that her son was missing out on the sort of close relationship she had had with her daughter when she was a baby. She finally spoke to her GP and asked for help. The GP, who had already prescribed antidepressants, referred her to a perinatal psychologist who was able to help her with the grieving process and to gradually make space in her mind and her day to enjoy and cherish her little boy.

Worrying that the baby doesn't love them

Parents who may have had difficult early lives may be over-sensitive to perceived 'rejection' by their baby. A mother feeling this way may say to a health professional, 'I don't think my baby likes me very much'.

This may be a result of either a misinterpretation of her baby's cues or a lack of sensitivity to her baby's attempts at emotional regulation (see Chapter 6 for more detail). For example, a baby who is over-stimulated may look away from his mother when she is trying (perhaps a little too hard) to make face-to-face contact with him. A sensitive mother who is feeling vulnerable in her role may interpret this as rejection. Similarly an older baby may no longer focus on his mother during a feed and may look all around the room instead. A mother with her own insecurities may feel unloved or no longer needed by her baby. These apparently small moments can be painful for some new mothers.

Some of the material in Underdown and Barlow (2012) *Maternal Emotional Wellbeing and Infant Development* and the new *Getting to Know your Baby* guidance for new parents developed by Warwick University (2014) (www.your-baby.org.uk) might help parents with these sorts of difficulties. The material for the latter is available as a smart-phone app. designed to promote emotional well-being before and after birth. It includes short videos introducing parents to observing their babies closely, including topics such as 'baby states' and 'early interactions'. The app can be personalised by new parents for their newborns.

Worrying about circumstances at home

Women who express concern or worry about the circumstances at home or about what they are taking their baby home to may be expressing one of many concerns. These could include:

- Worry about an abusive or violent partner.

- Worry about debt or difficulties with benefit payments.

- Worry about refugee status, legal status and achieving leave to remain.

- Worry about a family member who is using drugs.

- Worry about other children at home and her capacity to cope with caring for them and a new baby.

- Worry about difficulties that she has not disclosed prior to delivery, such as an anxiety disorder e.g. agoraphobia or OCD, which will make it difficult for her to look after her baby without practical or specialist help.

All of these difficulties will benefit from sensitive exploration rather than immediate reassurance, even if solutions are not immediately available. Making another appointment to talk about the issues further or setting up an appointment with another resource all show a woman that she has been heard and her concerns to do the best for her baby have been acknowledged, whatever the challenges in her life that may make this difficult.

Women who cause concern: Identifying when further intervention is needed

Working closely with mothers and babies can stir strong feelings in professionals and community workers providing their care. These feelings might include being very worried about a mother or a baby, feeling hopeless about a family's circumstances or feelings provoked by a mother's approach to self-care or the care of her baby. This section is intended to help professional carers identify when further intervention or action is needed for women and their babies who are causing concern. See also Chapter 6 and Chapter 12 for a useful discussion of the need for professional supervision.

Women who are tearful and distressed

Women who are tearful and seem distressed can be in very many different states in terms of their mental health. Being tearful after the drama of giving birth may represent emotions across the spectrum including: relief, joy, fear, pride, memory of earlier losses, exhaustion, elation and many more. Regular tearfulness some weeks after giving birth will most likely have a very different meaning.

Being able to comfortably spend time with women who are tearful without hurrying them to mop up their tears will be more fruitful. Slowing things down, tentatively exploring what might be behind the tears and hearing about previous sadness or fears for the future are an important part of postnatal and antenatal care.

Women who appear very anxious

Anxiety disorder is becoming recognised as a very common feature of the perinatal period (Hogg, 2013). Many women presenting with ante- or postnatal depression will also have symptoms of anxiety disorder. Of course it is also completely normal to be anxious about things in pregnancy, in the run up to birth and delivery and when taking on the care of a newborn for the first time. Women presenting with normal levels of anxiety will need support, information and the understanding of non-judgemental, experienced staff.

Women with anxiety disorders, either generalised anxiety disorder (GAD), agoraphobia or OCD will need more careful support and, potentially, referral to a perinatal mental health team or other psychological treatment resource (see Chapter 3 on assessment).

It is worth noting that women with high levels of anxiety may be irritable, defensive or aggressive and may also complain of physical symptoms such as feeling hot, having palpitations, feeling dizzy and having chest pain. It is important that these sorts of physical symptoms are not too readily dismissed as 'psychological'. In the confidential enquiry into maternal death (Oates & Cantwell, 2011) there were a number of cases where physical symptoms were attributed to mental health difficulties and serious medical conditions were missed. Nevertheless, it is important that the level of distress and anxiety shown by a woman taking responsibility for a newborn is adequately attended to.

Women who are talking or hinting about suicide or self-harm

Item 10 in the Edinburgh Postnatal Depression Scale (Cox *et al*, 1987) asks about whether a woman has had thoughts about harming herself. It can be a difficult question to ask. In the author's view it is not a good shortcut to ask a woman to fill it in as a self-report questionnaire alone in a side room or, worse still, in a busy and noisy clinic. In a clinic setting the EPDS works best as a structure of prompts in a guided conversation (see Chapter 3).

If you suspect that a pregnant woman or a new mother might be having suicidal feelings it is important to ask some questions to explore whether you might be right. Possible questions might be:

- Do you ever wish everything would just stop or that you could take yourself off somewhere far away?

- Are you having any thoughts that are scaring you?

- Do you ever think it would be better if you weren't here?

- Do you ever think your family would be better off without you?

If there are real concerns about a risk of self-harm then this sort of discussion should be followed up by an assessment by a woman's GP or by a mental health practitioner. If a woman is actively suicidal and has an articulated plan of how she would do it, she may need accompanying to A&E, urgent assessment by a perinatal or liaison psychiatrist and/or admission to a mother and baby unit.

Reviewing suicides in the CMACE triennial report, Oates and Cantwell (2011) note that there has been no significant reduction in maternal suicide within six months of delivery since 1997. Two groups of women feature in the report which are distinct from the risk pattern of suicide in the general population:

1. Over half of the women who died were older, married women in comfortable circumstances with a previous psychiatric history but who were well during pregnancy.

2. This is in contrast to the characteristics of mothers who were substance misusers who died either from suicide or other causes – these women were, in the main, young, single, unemployed and socially deprived.

The majority of mothers who die by suicide do not also kill their baby. However, sadly, during the writing of this volume, a mother in Bristol did commit suicide by violent means and her baby died with her. So despite the low statistics, a concern about suicide risk is also a concern about child protection.

Case example

Romina, a young Bulgarian woman with a strained relationship with her parents, had recently married a man from another faith and had taken comfort from her new religious beliefs and rituals. Her husband worked long hours in a restaurant and she was anxious at times during her pregnancy and did not have friends locally because they were moving frequently to pursue affordable housing in privately rented flats. When she first came to the UK she had suffered a serious sexual assault. She had felt desperately lonely and unsupported and had made a suicide attempt in the immediate aftermath. Halfway through her pregnancy she had some worrying abdominal cramps and was hospitalised overnight. In the middle of the night she felt hot and very anxious and she told the night staff that she felt so uncomfortable that she wanted to leave. The night staff, not knowing her full history, said that it was impossible for her to leave at night because it was not safe. In the event she stuck it out on the ward but she later told a health worker who had got to know her that she had nearly left the ward alone in the middle of the night because of how desperate she had felt.

Women who express odd ideas or beliefs

Women's experience of pregnancy and giving birth is often one of the most vivid and stimulating times of their life. Women report powerful sensations, emotions, ideas and experiences. However for some women this powerful experience tips into something where their connection with reality is fractured. This is the experience of puerperal psychosis or postpartum psychosis (see Chapter 9 'Severe perinatal mental health difficulties'). Women may have disturbing or persecutory beliefs about themselves and their babies which can place both them and their baby at risk. Women may say they are not themselves and may hold the belief that their baby has a special identity, such as the devil or the messiah. Puerperal psychosis is a medical emergency because she may act on some of her disturbed psychotic beliefs. Because a woman's mental state can deteriorate rapidly, she will need urgent medical intervention from a psychiatrist.

Women who appear very detached from or disinterested in their baby

How a woman refers to her baby or the way she describes her baby's personality or behaviour is often something that stops a care worker or professional in their tracks. A mother might say 'Oh, he's got a temper on him alright' about a baby who is only weeks old.

This is referred to as the mother's 'representation' of her infant. This representation gives healthcare staff important information about the mother's thinking and about the emotional environment she is providing for her baby. Outcomes for babies whose mothers have negative representations of them are less favourable than those whose mothers see them more positively (Meins, 2013). If mothers are overtly negative about their babies or make hostile comments about their nature or behaviour, the attachment relationship to the baby, and hence his or her emotional care, is likely to be at risk. Referral to parent-infant services, and in more extreme cases social services, will be indicated.

Women who seem preoccupied with their own needs and appear unable to prioritise their baby's needs

Similarly, where mothers appear preoccupied with other issues, such as their own body, their relationship with the baby's father or other male partner, their pursuit of alcohol or other substances and seem unable to keep the baby's needs in mind, optimal care for the baby is at risk and safeguarding concerns may need to be raised (see case example of Leanne in Chapter 6).

Vulnerability factors for the development of ante and postnatal depression

Pregnancy, giving birth and early motherhood are a challenge for all women. But for a significant number of women the difficulties can result in ante and/or postnatal depression or other maternal mental health difficulties (See Chapter 10). Below are some of the key factors that make perinatal depression and other difficulties more likely to emerge.

- A pre-existing depression, before pregnancy or antenatally.
- A poor attachment pattern in her own childhood e.g. distant, critical, neglectful or abusive parenting.
- Marital or relationship difficulties.
- Lack of practical support from her partner or others.
- Lack of a confiding relationship.
- Death of a parent before age 11.
- Experience of physical or sexual abuse in childhood or early sexual relationships.

- Major life events during pregnancy or after the birth e.g. moving house, relationship breakdown, job loss, bereavement or major illness in the family.

- Previous perinatal losses e.g. still birth, miscarriage, cot death.

- Unexpected difficulties with the baby e.g. instrumental delivery, baby needing special care, 'traumatic' delivery.

- Mother herself ill post-delivery.

These factors can be grouped under five broad headings highlighting different areas of vulnerability.

Psychosocial history

A difficult relationship with her own mother is often a factor in maternal depression. Where women have experienced physical or sexual abuse in childhood this is even more likely. In psychological terms these experiences involve loss; the loss of childhood but also, crucially, self-esteem. For women losing a parent in childhood, mothering their own children is always coloured with the loss of their own parent.

Current social circumstances

Women who have little social and practical support, for example young single mothers, may be vulnerable to depression. If they do not have access to a confiding relationship the experience of caring for a young baby can feel very isolating. Recent life events such as moving house, becoming homeless or coming to another country as a refugee all increase the risk of anxiety and depression. Depression among women suffering domestic violence is very common and pregnancy is a known risk factor for escalation of such violence.

Mental health history

Women who have had previous mental illness at other points in their life will have a greater risk of antenatal and postnatal mental health difficulties. Women who have previously suffered from a severe perinatal mental illness, such as severe depression or postpartum psychosis, have a high risk of further difficulty with a subsequent pregnancy (around 50%). If there has been an episode of severe perinatal illness in a first degree relative (mother or sister) in a woman's family this will increase her own risk of becoming ill (NICE, 2014).

It is helpful to ask women if they have ever needed treatment, counselling or hospital admission for mental health conditions such as depression, anxiety disorder, bipolar disorder or psychosis. A history of problems with drugs or alcohol is also significant.

Childbearing history

Previous childbearing loss, including earlier abortions, stillbirths and miscarriages, create a vulnerability for maternal mental health difficulties. These experiences can create anxiety and doubt about safely delivering a healthy baby and complicate the new pregnancy with feelings of anger, guilt and sadness.

Role adjustment

While society colours images of motherhood with a positive hue, women themselves have to negotiate a number of losses as part of their adjustment to motherhood. For working women, motherhood involves a shifting identity where both status and income are lost as a woman leaves her place of work. For all women, her relationships with family, friends and her partner have to accommodate change. For women who have enjoyed feeling in control of their lives and/or like to feel independent and not ask for help from others, motherhood can powerfully challenge their sense of self.

Summary of contributing factors

1. Social factors, such as financial stresses, housing problems and noisy or aggressive neighbours can contribute to the development of depression.

2. Negative views and judgements about the self contribute to feelings of depression.

3. Early childhood experience, especially the loss of a parent before the age of 11 and neglectful or abusive parenting, increase the likelihood of depression in adulthood.

4. Women without a supportive partner or other confiding relationship (such as a mother, sister, or a close friend) are more likely to become depressed than women who do.

This last point is the basis of many first level interventions for perinatal mental health difficulties. For example, listening visits, which may be provided by health visitors and family nurses, provide the same empathic support and containment of anxiety that more fortunate women may be able to access from their own social network. All four points together are very helpful to bear in mind when offering help to women and planning care pathways and services to support them.

References

Cox JL, Holden JM & Sagovsky R (1987) Detection of postnatal depression. Development of the 10-item Edinburgh Postnatal Depression Scale. *British Journal of Psychiatry* **150** (6) 782–786.

Department of Health (2013) *Health Visiting: the voice of service users. Learning from service users' experiences to inform the development of UK health visiting practice and services* [online]. National Nursing Research Unit, King's College London. Available at: https://www.kcl.ac.uk/nursing/research/nnru/publications/Reports/Voice-of-service-user-report-July-2013-FINAL.pdf (accessed April 2016).

Hogg S (2013) *Prevention in Mind. All Babies Count: Spotlight on perinatal mental health* [online]. NSPCC. Available at: http://www.nspcc.org.uk/globalassets/documents/research-reports/all-babies-count-spotlight-perinatal-mental-health.pdf (accessed April 2016).

Meins E (2013) Sensitive attunement to infants' internal states: operationalizing the construct of mind-mindedness. *Attachment and Human Development* **15** (5-6) 524–544.

NICE (2014) *Antenatal and Postnatal Mental Health: Clinical management and service guidance* [online]. Available at: https://www.nice.org.uk/guidance/cg192/resources/guidance-antenatal-and-postnatal-mental-health-clinical-management-and-service-guidance.pdf (accessed April 2016).

Oates M & Cantwell R (2011) Deaths from psychiatric causes. In: Centre for Maternal and Child Enquiries (CMACE) Saving Mothers' Lives: Reviewing Maternal Deaths To Make Motherhood Safer: 2006-08. *BJOG* **118** (S1) 1–203.

Parker R (2005) *Torn in Two: The experience of maternal ambivalence*. London: Virago.

Underdown A & Barlow J (2012) *Maternal Emotional Wellbeing and Infant Development: A good practice guide for midwives* [online]. Royal College of Midwives. Available at: https://www.rcm.org.uk/sites/default/files/Emotional%20Wellbeing_Guide_WEB.pdf (accessed May 2016).

Warwick University (2014) *Getting to Know your Baby* [online]. Available at: www.your-baby.org.uk (accessed April 2016).

Chapter 6: Keeping the baby in mind: baby-mindedness in parents and professionals

Eleanor Grant

Introduction

There is now overwhelming research evidence from the fields of neuroscience, child development and psychotherapy to suggest that the first few months and years of life are crucial in laying down the foundations for future emotional and social functioning. This chapter will give an overview of some of the relevant concepts, including attachment, and the importance of 'keeping the baby in mind'. It will discuss the impact on attachment of postnatal depression and other difficulties, including childhood abuse. It will also introduce new clinical services that aim to support the attachment relationship. For midwives and health visitors, increased awareness of the emerging attachment relationship can help inform professional practice.

The everyday drama of childbirth brings a new chapter in the lives of the mother, her partner, her family and her baby. New relationships are brought into being and existing ones transformed. Pregnancy and delivery can bring great hope and excitement but can also stir anxieties and unexpected fears. The intense emotions around this time can be turbulent and sometimes overwhelming. How a new mother negotiates this time of change will depend on many factors, including what support she has (partner, family, professional) and her own experience of being parented.

The early weeks and months of life are unremembered, and yet neuroscience and psychotherapy research demonstrates how crucially significant this time is in shaping the individual's development (see Gerhardt, 2015, for an overview). For the baby to develop well, the environment needs to be good enough. The infant's relationship with his main carer, usually his mother initially, and later his father too, forms the environment in which he grows and which affects the development of the brain and endocrine system. The brain adapts to the situation the baby finds himself in by developing connections in response to the stimulation it receives. Repeated experience reinforces connections until the pathways are 'hardwired' into the brain, changing the basic brain architecture.

The baby's first relationships will therefore influence his expectations for all subsequent relationships, including those with professionals. The emotional environment of the parent-infant relationship will influence how self-control, emotional regulation, and response to threat and stress develop. The baby is not merely the passive recipient of care, however, but an active participant in the unfolding scenario with his parents. Babies are born to be social (see Murray & Andrews, 2000) and from birth seek to engage with their caregivers. A new baby needs his caregivers to keep him alive and to help him make sense of and manage the world and his own emotions. How the attachment relationship develops with the primary caregiver (usually the mother) will depend on how sensitively she responds to the baby and how attuned she is to his needs. Sensitive and attuned responsive care offers the optimal foundation for healthy development. What the baby learns to expect from others will influence his way of being in the world and whether he can expect to rely on others to manage distress.

Containment

Caregivers are involved in holding the baby together physically: keeping him fed, clothed and held. Holding and physical containment is vital (a new baby can feel frightened by having his clothes removed and may be quieted by being wrapped up again) but being 'held' emotionally is equally important. A tiny baby can be overwhelmed by his intense emotions without help from another. He relies on the caregiver to tolerate and modify distress. A parent who can hear and understand his distress and who is not overwhelmed can offer him a way of making it more bearable. This kind of containment, as described by Bion (1962), offers emotional support in the here and now, and communicates that such feelings can be survived and managed. The mother's capacity to tolerate the communicated emotion renders it less overwhelming for the baby. This is the beginnings of emotional regulation and a foundation for secure attachment. In a parallel process, professionals working with families are often called upon to help contain the seemingly overwhelming emotions of the parents. This containing function can help the mother process her own emotions and restore the capacity to think. In a further parallel, the supervision process offers containment to the worker. The regularity and reliability of supervision is important in maintaining a safe place to explore and think about the work (see Chapter 12). The offer of regular supervision means the worker does not have to 'hold' the issues alone and can talk through and reflect on any concerns. Knowing that there is a supervision session coming up can allow the professional to contain the worries until that time. In the same way that a child, when faced with pressure or stress, might remember a loving parent or grandparent encouraging them, professionals can rely on a supervision space for support. This space can reduce anxiety and restore the capacity to think about the issues rather than be overwhelmed by them. This increased confidence is then transmitted in turn to the families the professional works with.

Case example: containment

Leanne was visited by her health visitor who was concerned that she was depressed. She had her own one bedroom flat but since the birth of her baby boy she had hardly spent any time there. She said she needed help clearing up the boxes of stuff that were taking up too much space in her flat. She had more or less broken up with the father of her son and did not like to go out with the baby on her own. When the health visitor visited, Leanne told her she had lost her purse and this was creating money difficulties for her. At the next visit she spent a long time telling the health visitor how she could not decide what to ask her parents to buy her for her birthday. At both appointments her baby son was apparently asleep in his buggy. The health visitor was aware that Leanne seemed to need a lot of looking after herself and it seemed very hard to make a space for Leanne's son's needs to get much of a look in.

The health visitor went away feeling frustrated and a bit useless. She wanted to support Leanne but she also wanted to try and keep the baby in mind – which was hard with Leanne's constant talk about other issues. It seemed Leanne needed distraction from both the boxes in the flat and the other 'stuff' that she felt was dragging her down.

The health visitor discussed her own feelings in supervision. She realised that she was the one holding the concern for the baby and that she felt irritated and inadequate by the difficulty she had in helping Leanne think about her son's needs. Supervision helped disentangle what belonged to the health visitor and what belonged with Leanne. It seemed that Leanne had communicated very effectively how inadequate she felt and how she felt she did not get enough support from her family. The health visitor was able to return to the situation and not feel overwhelmed by frustration and feeling useless. As the visits progressed the baby, encouraged by Leanne with the health visitor's support, began to be a more active presence in the room.

Attachment

Attachment theory originates in the work of John Bowlby (1969, 1988) who described attachment in evolutionary terms as important for the infant's survival. The caregiver's presence is also important in helping the infant regulate emotions and develop a feeling of security. So attachment is about keeping safe and secure, physically and psychologically, when threatened with stress and distress. Attachment behaviour, such as seeking proximity to the caregiver, will be elicited when under stress. The infant's capacity for self-control, emotional regulation, and his response to threat and stress is learned in the context of the attachment relationship.

Facilitating circumstances

In good enough conditions the parents' sensitive, responsive care will help promote resilience and adaptability in the infant which forms the foundation of robust mental health. The experiences are internalised and inform an individual's expectations of the world and themselves.

Secure attachment

When the caregiving is good enough, when the mother is sensitive and responsive and well attuned to her baby's needs, the infant learns to rely on the parent to provide security and comfort and will develop a secure attachment. He develops a mental representation of the caregiver as reliable and of himself as lovable and worthy of care. In time the growing child will be able to use the parent as a secure base from which to explore and as a safe haven and place of comfort to return to. The infant takes this advantage with him into adulthood.

Case example: secure attachment

Robert's mother was able to respond sensitively to his needs and not become overwhelmed or feel persecuted. She was able to contain his emotions and think about what was going on for him and what he needed. Being able to mentalise and reflect on her own emotional states, as well as his, allowed her to see his emotions as communications and respond to his needs. This helped Robert learn that he could rely on his mother to comfort him and help him manage his distress. Once comforted, Robert was able to resume exploration and play.

Babies in less favourable circumstances

When the baby's experience of his parent does not bring the expectation that his needs will be met, a different mental representation will develop: attachment will not be secure. Insecurely attached infants will not be able to use the caregiver in the same way to soothe their aroused emotions. They may end up either over-regulating themselves (playing down distress) or under-regulating themselves (playing up distress), or both, in an attempt to manage overwhelming emotion. This, again, will form a pattern or expectation regarding future relationships.

Mary Ainsworth (1978) and her colleagues elaborated Bowlby's theory and categorised attachment as secure, insecure-avoidant or insecure-ambivalent. She developed the procedure known as the Strange Situation to categorise infant attachment behaviour. This research procedure involves two brief separations from the caregiver. The infant's behaviour during separation and especially on reunion with the caregiver formed the basis of the classification into originally three, later four, categories of attachment.

Avoidant attachment

In avoidant attachment the infant learns to play down emotion, especially distress. Ainsworth noted that the mothers of avoidant infants often appeared to be emotionally unavailable to their babies, rigid and rejecting of the baby's distress. A baby in this circumstance might begin to expect that his emotional needs will not be met and so learns over time to manage his emotions on his own. He over-regulates his emotion, not letting any distress show. The baby may appear to be content, with his behaviour resembling independent play, but this may in fact represent a dismissing of his own needs with a focus on play as a distraction.

Case example: avoidant attachment

Jayden's mother always found it hard to hold him close. She seemed to find it difficult to respond to his need for physical proximity. This made it hard for her to comfort him when he needed it and she appeared to reject his attempts to get close to her. She tried to jolly him along when he cried, distracting him with a toy or a new object, and seemed not to register his distress. It could be that this is what she had learned from her own upbringing about how to deal with distress. In time, Jayden looked less and less to his mother for comfort and seemed to suppress his urge to seek proximity to her when he was upset; he learned to manage his distress on his own. He would not look to his mother for comfort but focused on exploration.

Ambivalent attachment

In ambivalent attachment the caregiver offers an insufficient or inconsistent response. The infant becomes highly vigilant and tends to heighten rather than downplay his attachment needs. He displays clingy vigilance, intensifying his own distress until he becomes inconsolable, while continuing to seek solace. He both seeks and rejects care, leaving him feeling frustrated and distressed.

Case example: ambivalent attachment

Olivia's mother seemed overwhelmed by any display of distress and responded inconsistently, at times trying to comfort her and at other times finding this too demanding. She appeared preoccupied with her own issues and often panicked when Olivia was upset, leaving them both in a state of agitation. Olivia became increasingly uncertain about what reaction to expect from her mother and tended to be watchful and clingy but not easily comforted. This inhibited her ability to explore.

Disorganised attachment

A fourth category was later described by Mary Main (Main & Solomon, 1986; 1990) as disorganised attachment. She suggested that infants in these cases displayed an incoherent lack of ability to use any consistent strategy to manage their stress on separation. It was thought that these infants had had experience of a frightening caregiver, so when comfort or reassurance was sought the infant was placed in an impossible conflict between seeking care from the caregiver and avoiding them as the source of distress.

Case example: disorganised attachment

For Catherine, relying on her mother for solace was fraught with difficulty, as her mother was often the source of her distress. Catherine's mother was not able to be aware of Catherine's needs. She had an unsettled background with a history of abuse and unresolved trauma. Her efforts to manage her difficult experiences had led to problems with alcohol and drugs. This meant she was unable to look after Catherine in the way she would have wanted. She experienced her daughter's needs as frighteningly demanding and she often responded by becoming angry. This was terrifying for Catherine, as her mother could not manage or regulate her own emotional states and was therefore not available to help Catherine with hers. Catherine found it hard to concentrate or be engaged in any activity and was easily flipped into inconsistent, panicky responses herself. She did not appear to have a coherent strategy for managing distress.

Patricia Crittenden (2008), in a further development, suggested that infants categorised as displaying 'disorganised' attachment behaviours could actually be seen to be using highly organised strategies developed to keep themselves safe in the face of unpredictable, frightened and frightening attachment figures. In Crittenden's model the main organising factor is danger, with attachment behaviour being the strategies infants develop in order to protect themselves from this danger. She suggested that in these circumstances a distressed infant may learn to inhibit displays of emotion – crying for example, as crying might bring an angry response from the parent. In this scenario the infant performs the regulatory function for the parent, that is, adapts behaviour in order to 'look after' the adult. In adulthood we may be able to support another person's emotional regulation but in infancy the baby or child does not have the emotional maturity to cope with this. The impact of this early burden may last into adulthood.

Researchers have demonstrated (see, for example, Fonagy *et al*, 1991; Iyengar *et al*, 2014) that there is a significant correspondence between a parent's attachment style – that is, the pattern of attachment to their own parents (George *et al*, 1985) – and that of their offspring: securely attached parents tend to have children who are securely attached to them. The parent's early experiences and how she (or he) thinks about them will affect the way she parents her own baby.

Baby-mindedness, reflective function and mentalising

The development of secure attachment is predicated on the parent being accessible, interpreting the baby's communications accurately and responding appropriately. This sensitivity is mediated by the ability of the parent to treat the infant as a separate being, an individual with a mind of his own. A mother can be said to be baby-minded when she can think about the baby's internal states, 'tune in' to the baby's feelings and understand the baby's behaviour in light of this: she can 'keep the baby in mind'. A capacity for reflective function (recognising that people have mental states that inform their behaviour) enables a process of mentalisation, where people (oneself and others) can be understood in terms of feelings, desires and so on. This enables the parent to be curious about what the infant might be thinking or feeling; she can wonder about the baby's internal states. In this way the infant is helped to feel understood. He is supported to develop his own sense of himself and his feelings, through being held in mind by another who makes sense of his feelings for him and helps him manage them. Mentalisation is therefore important in the beginnings of emotional regulation in the infant and in making behaviour more understandable and predictable for the parent. A mother who can understand her baby's cries in terms of the baby needing comfort rather than because he is randomly making a fuss or intending to 'get at' her is more able to tolerate another broken night's sleep despite her own exhaustion.

Elizabeth Meins (2013) has elaborated the concept of 'mind-mindedness'. Maternal mind-mindedness is the mother's ability to interpret her infant's thoughts and feelings and comment appropriately, giving voice to the baby's intentions. This capacity to view the child as a mental agent has been shown to predict sensitive and responsive parenting behaviour. When the mother accurately identifies and names the infant's feelings, this forms the basis for the growing child to begin to identify his own feelings and think about them. A mother, attending her crying infant, may wonder about the baby's experience and verbalise her response: 'Oh, it sounds like you're really uncomfortable; perhaps you're hungry? Would you like a feed? Or maybe you need a nappy change. Yes, look, you're all wet, you poor thing. Let's get you a clean nappy. Come on, little one.' In time the child grows to understand that other people have feelings too. This paves the way for co-operative and loving relationships throughout life, based on self-confidence and empathy for others.

Both mentalisation and mind-mindedness can be impacted by stress. Threat reduces the capacity to mentalise and, conversely, being able to mentalise may help reduce parental stress by making the infant's behaviour more understandable. Parents who have low reflective function may be more likely to view the baby's needs and responses as negative or even persecutory, based on a belief that the baby deliberately wants to punish them: 'She's crying because she doesn't like me'. A vicious circle can be established where the mother feels stressed by the baby's behaviour and this makes her less able to reflect on her own and the baby's feelings. Reflecting on emotional states can also be painful and at times overwhelming. A mother struggling to respond to her baby's needs may need support herself to develop her capacity for reflective function.

Case example: Martha

Martha struggled when her first child was born. As a successful professional leading a team, she was used to making decisions and feeling in control. She did not feel in control once her son was born. Her own mother had died some years before and she felt overwhelmed by the relentless pressures of new motherhood. At times she thought that the baby was 'out to get her' and that she would never be able to satisfy his needs. She believed that other mothers found it easy to look after their babies. She began to feel frustrated and cross with the baby, which heightened her guilt. Her husband noticed how pressured she seemed and asked about how she was feeling. Martha was able to talk to her husband about how much more difficult it was than she had expected and how much she missed her mother now that she had had a baby herself. Her husband understood how vulnerable she felt and was able to support her. Being able to talk about and reflect on her own needs as well as those of the baby helped Martha acknowledge difficult feelings and respond to her baby in a sensitive way.

Effects of maternal mental health on attachment

For most mothers, the transition to parenthood proceeds with a mixture of excitement, apprehensiveness and anticipation, which they navigate with the help and support of those around them. Ideally, the relationship with the baby and keeping the baby in mind will begin during the pregnancy. As the foetus grows and begins to take up more space, the mother also begins to make 'space' for the infant in her world, both physically and psychologically. Her capacity for this will be related to her own experience of being parented and her own mental health.

A mother's mental health will be impacted by many factors, including her own attachment status, her material circumstances (eg. poverty/housing issues) and the support she has. These many factors will influence how available the mother is to her baby emotionally and how sensitive she is able to be. A mother who is consumed by her own issues or who is very depressed may well miss her baby's cues or misinterpret them. Vulnerability in the infant can seem unsettling or even frightening for a mother. She can lose her capacity to respond to her baby in a way that validates his actions and desire for a relationship with her.

Impact of the parent's own history

In her seminal paper *Ghosts in the nursery*, Selma Fraiberg famously stated: 'In every nursery there are ghosts. They are the visitors from the unremembered past of the parents, the uninvited guests at the christening' (Fraiberg *et al*, 1975). In this very readable account of her work at the Child Development Project at the University of Michigan, Fraiberg described the difficulties some parents have with unresolved trauma, which can, unwittingly, be recreated in the relationship with the baby. Pregnancy and new parenthood can put us in touch with our own experience of being parented and traumatic early experience can be re-awakened during this time. Fraiberg suggested that when a parent's early childhood experiences were frightening or neglectful, the internal world of the parent may cloud their ability to respond sensitively to their infant and thus impair the quality of the parent-infant relationship. In this way trauma can be passed from one generation to the next. Fraiberg's early work has inspired and informed the development of infant mental health services ever since.

Not all parents with a history of cruelty, neglect or other trauma will necessarily bring this to bear on the infant, as Fraiberg points out. As in fairy tales, there may be forces for good at work that mitigate the impact of the more malevolent 'ghosts'. Lieberman and her colleagues (2005) suggest that benevolent early experiences can be equally potent and helpful in fostering positive, loving parent-child relationships. They argue that these 'angels in the nursery' can be channelled to protect against adversity and even overwhelming trauma. If there are enough early nurturing experiences, these can offer protection, hope and an alternative model of relationship. For most of us the ghosts and angels will coexist in dynamic balance and the outcome will be good enough. Having the experience of being known, loved and understood promotes security and can be protective even in traumatic circumstances. A child who, despite unfavourable circumstances, can access instances of connection and positive emotional experience with a caring adult can develop confidence and the ability to be effective in the world. The influence of a loving grandparent who can offer the shared experience of emotional connection or a sensitive, encouraging teacher who believes in the child can help mitigate the negative influences of a difficult home situation.

A woman's history can affect not only her parenting but also the experience of childbirth. Mothers who have been sexually abused in childhood may approach childbirth with trepidation and can sometimes be re-traumatised by their experiences. Women with histories of abuse can easily feel out of control and unable to trust those around them, which can increase their difficulties during childbirth. Many women will not disclose, even when asked, that they have suffered sexual abuse, but will maintain silence, which can present difficulties for those caring for them (Montgomery *et al*, 2015). Midwives will therefore not necessarily know who has experienced childhood abuse. Services need to be respectful, compassionate and sensitive to all women in their care, in order to maintain the dignity of all and reduce the likelihood of childbirth being traumatic for the mother.

There may be other experiences that can affect a mother's capacity to respond sensitively to her baby. Poverty, mental health problems, domestic violence, migration from homeland and family, and disability in parent or child can all make parenting more difficult. A significant minority of new mothers (around 10–15%) are depressed postnatally. Maternal depression and anxiety often go together and frequently start during pregnancy. Post-traumatic stress can also impinge on the mother-infant relationship (Bauer *et al*, 2014); mothers who have had traumatic experiences can find that their baby's distress acts as a trigger for their own traumatic distress response.

Supporting the attachment relationship and baby-mindedness

Not every mother who experiences depression will have a difficult or damaging relationship with her baby. Similarly, mothers with other mental health issues can be supported to optimise their relationships with their infants so as to minimise later attachment difficulties: adverse effects are not inevitable.

Fraiberg and her colleagues pioneered a way of working with parents and infants together, which became known as the Fraiberg Intervention Model (Fraiberg, 1980; Shapiro, 2009). This way of working focused on the mother-infant relationship and used the relationship between the parent and the professional as the vehicle. It became the model for many subsequent parent-infant services in the US and the UK. The capacity for the worker to contain the mother's emotional distress enabled the mother to respond more fully to her baby. As Fraiberg put it:

'When the mother's own cries are heard, she will hear her child's cries.'
(Fraiberg *et al*, 1975, p396)

This was found to be particularly helpful for parents who had suffered abuse or trauma as children. In this optimistic approach the worker also held the baby in mind and wondered, out loud, what the baby might be experiencing and feeling as the mother interacted with him. This 'speaking for the baby' enhanced the mother's capacity for reflection and mentalising, which enriched the mother-infant relationship. Wondering out loud what the baby is experiencing or commenting on the infant's response to a situation can bring his experience alive for his mother: 'I wonder whether he feels a bit uncertain coming into this unfamiliar room,' or, 'You like it when Mummy bangs the drum with you, don't you?' In this way the baby is considered as a person in his own right, with his own feelings, which are being thought about. Keeping the father in mind too, even when he is absent, is also important, as he will be a presence, if only in the mother's mind.

Helping new mothers and fathers to think about the myriad emotional experiences of becoming a parent, including the difficult aspects, can be hard work. Keeping alert to the experiences of all parties (the infant, the parents – and oneself) in the moment can be challenging. Reflective supervision and the increasing literature focusing compassionately on parents' and babies' emotional lives – such as *Finding Your Way with Your Baby* (Daws & de Rementeria, 2015), which brings together insights from years of professional experience and recent research – can help support this rewarding work.

Services supporting the parent-infant relationship

Midwives and health visitors see women throughout pregnancy and the postnatal period (and beyond). This offers an opportunity to observe and support the developing attachment relationship and to model baby-mindedness. There may be difficulties that start in pregnancy; for example, depression in the postnatal period is frequently preceded by antenatal depression. Attachment problems can start to become apparent even before the baby is born and may need to be handled sensitively.

Postnatally, mothers may need support in adapting to the new circumstances and in being compassionate to themselves. Many different cultures enshrine an idealised view of motherhood, which can make it hard for new mothers to feel 'good enough'. Midwives and health visitors can help by acknowledging how common the fears and concerns of new mothers are. Thoughts and feelings that are frequently unacknowledged or avoided as too difficult can be allowed expression in a thoughtful, trusting relationship with a sensitive professional. Motherhood is not all easy, joyous feelings: ambivalence about the baby is very common and not unhealthy (Parker, 2005).

For a decade and more there has been a growing awareness of the need for more relationship-focused services (Balbernie, 2002). Many recent service developments in the care of pregnant and postnatal mothers are designed around the parent-infant relationship. The evidence suggests that skilled professionals with appropriate training and supervision are able to develop supportive relationships with parents, which can in turn enhance the parent-infant relationship (see the Sutton Trust's 2014 report *Baby Bonds* for an overview). Those programmes which involved fathers were found to be especially effective.

In the UK there are many programmes that aim to support the development of reflective parenting and thus promote attachment security and emotional development. These include the following:

- **The Antenatal and Postnatal Promotional Guides** (Day *et al*, 2014) are widely used by health visitors in the UK and help promote reflective function and relationship with the unborn, and later, newborn baby. The guides offer a structured but flexible and consistent approach to engaging and supporting parents through the transition to parenthood and the baby's early development.

- **The Solihull Approach**, originally devised for health visitors for children with sleep difficulties, brings together the concepts of containment, reciprocity and behaviour management (Douglas & Ginty, 2001). The approach trains professionals to work reflectively with families and offers parenting courses directly to families.

- **The Family Nurse Partnership (FNP)** originates from work in America and offers intensive support to vulnerable teenage first time mothers. Specially trained FNP nurses visit mothers regularly from early pregnancy until the child's second birthday.

- **The Minding the Baby project** in Glasgow, Sheffield and York also originates from work in America. It involves home visiting from the seventh month of pregnancy until the child is two years old. Both FNP and Minding the Baby have demonstrated improved outcomes for parent and child.

- **The Circle of Security programme**, also from America, is a relationship-based early intervention program designed to enhance attachment security between parents and children. The Circle of Security graphic (see Figure 6.1 on p90) represents the basic tenets of the programme in a memorable way. It shows the hands of the parent offering a secure base from which the child feels confident to explore, leaving the parent, who he knows will be there to watch over and delight in him – 'Look at me, Mummy!' – and offering a safe haven that welcomes return and brings comfort and soothing after the excitement of exploration.

- **Mellow Parenting and Mellow Babies**, for the under-ones, are courses designed to support families where a relationship difficulty with a small child is identified. The approach was designed in Scotland for highly vulnerable and stressed families. It has been shown to engage hard to reach families and to enhance mother-child interactions (Puckering *et al*, 1994; 2010).

- **Infant massage** is a 'hands-on' intervention which has been shown to support the parent-infant relationship. By bringing the parent and baby together through touch, it can deepen their relationship.

- **Video Interaction Guidance (VIG)** is used increasingly by health visitors to help scaffold positive interactions between parent and infant. It is a collaborative relationship-based intervention, which uses video clips of parent-baby interaction to reflect on the relationship and how to develop it by enhancing communication between parent and baby.

- **Wait, Watch and Wonder** is a play-based psychotherapeutic approach that encourages parents to follow their child's lead. This child-led approach helps promote positive relationships by enhancing parental sensitivity and responsiveness through supporting reflection on the child's experience and feelings.

- **Parent-Infant Psychotherapy** might be appropriate where more intensive intervention is required, for example, where the mother's early experience has left her with unresolved trauma that interferes with her capacity to bond with her baby. Parent-infant psychotherapy is available from some specialist perinatal and infant mental health services, such as those provided by the Parent Infant Partnership (PIP) UK programmes.

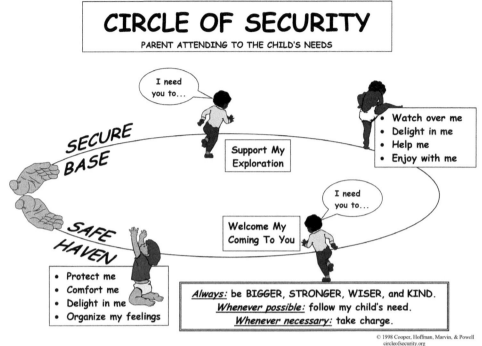

Figure 6.1: The Circle of Security. Reprinted with permission from Cooper G, Hoffman K, Marvin, R & Powell, B (1998) *Circle of Security: Parent attending to the child's needs.*

Further information on various programmes across the UK can be found in Jane Barlow and P. O. Svanberg's book *Keeping the Baby in Mind: Infant mental health in practice* (Barlow & Svanberg, 2009).

All these approaches are designed to help develop baby-mindedness in the parent and support the mother (and the family) to enjoy the baby. Working with families and the intense emotions surrounding childbirth and parenting can be exhilarating but also exhausting and difficult to contain. When professionals are under pressure, the risk of falling back on meeting service needs rather than keeping the baby in mind in the care you provide is much greater (Menzies Lyth, 1960). Regular reflective supervision is vital in order to offer the holding environment necessary for the worker to continue to contain the emotional content of the work and fully hold the mother and baby in mind.

Conclusion

The importance of the early years in infant development is increasingly acknowledged. Good maternal mental health will contribute to good infant mental health. The attachment relationships that the baby forms will establish the blueprint for later relationships and will affect the capacity for emotional regulation. Parents' own stories and experiences of being parented will, of course, impact on their capacity to attend to their baby and hear his cries. Over-stressed or traumatised parents will find it harder to focus on their baby's needs, but parental baby-mindedness, mentalisation and reflective function can all be supported through sensitive, responsive services.

References

Ainsworth MDS, Blehar MC, Waters E & Wall S (1978) *Patterns of Attachment: A psychological study of the Strange Situation*. Hillsdale, NJ: Erlbaum.

Balbernie R (2002) *An Infant Mental Health Service: The importance of the early years and evidence-based practice*. London: Child Psychotherapy Trust.

Barlow J & Svanberg PO (Eds) (2009) *Keeping the Baby in Mind: Infant mental health in practice*. London: Routledge.

Bauer A, Parsonage M, Knapp M, Iemmi V & Adelaja B (2014) *The Costs of Perinatal Mental Health Problems*. London: Centre for Mental Health.

Bion WR (1962) *Learning from Experience*. New York: Basic Books.

Bowlby J (1969) *Attachment*. London: Pelican.

Bowlby J (1988) *A Secure Base: Clinical applications of attachment theory*. London: Routledge.

Cooper G, Hoffman K, Marvin, R & Powell, B (1998) *Circle of Security: Parent attending to the child's needs* [online]. Available at: http://circleofsecurity.net/wp-content/uploads/2012/02/COS_chart-childsneeds.pdf (accessed April 2016).

Crittenden PM (2008) *Raising Parents: Attachment, parenting and child safety*. Cullompton: Willan Publishing.

Daws D & de Rementeria A (2015) *Finding Your Way with Your Baby*. Hove: Routledge.

Day C, Morton A, Ibbeson A, Maddison S, Pease R & Smith K (2014) Antenatal/postnatal promotional guide: evidence-based intervention. *Journal of Health Visiting* **2** (12) 658–669.

Douglas H & Ginty M (2001) The Solihull Approach: changes in health visiting practice. *Community Practitioner* **74** (6) 222–224.

Fonagy P, Steele H & Steele M (1991) Maternal representations of attachment during pregnancy predict the organization of infant-mother attachment at one year of age. *Child Development* **62** 891–905.

Fraiberg S (Ed) (1980) *Clinical Studies in Infant Mental Health: The first year of life*. London: Tavistock.

Fraiberg S, Adelson E & Shapiro V (1975) Ghosts in the nursery: a psychoanalytic approach to the problems of impaired infant-mother relationships. *Journal of the American Academy of Child Psychiatry* **14** (3) 387–421.

George C, Kaplan N & Main M (1985) *The Adult Attachment Interview* [unpublished manuscript]. Berkeley, CA: University of California.

Gerhardt S (2015) *Why Love Matters: How affection shapes a baby's brain* (2nd edition). Hove: Routledge.

Iyengar U, Kim S, Martinez S, Fonagy P & Strathearn L (2014) Unresolved trauma in mothers: intergenerational effects and the role of reorganization. *Frontiers in Psychology* **5** (Article 966) [online]. Available at: http://journal.frontiersin.org/article/10.3389/fpsyg.2014.00966/full (accessed April 2016).

Lieberman AF, Padrón E, van Horn P & Harris WW (2005) Angels in the nursery: the intergenerational transmission of benevolent parental influences. *Infant Mental Health Journal* **26** (6) 504–520.

Main M & Solomon J (1986) Discovery of a new, insecure-disorganized/disoriented attachment pattern. In: TB Brazelton and M Yogman (Eds) *Affective Development in Infancy* (pp 95–124). Norwood, NJ: Ablex.

Main M & Solomon J (1990) Procedures for identifying disorganized/disoriented infants during the Ainsworth Strange Situation. In: M Greenberg, D Cicchetti and EM Cummings (Eds) *Attachment in the Preschool Years* (pp121–160).Chicago, IL: University of Chicago Press.

Meins E (2013) Sensitive attunement to infants' internal states: operationalizing the construct of mind-mindedness. *Attachment & Human Development* **15** (5–6) 524–544.

Menzies Lyth I (1960) Social systems as a defense against anxiety: an empirical study of the nursing service of a general hospital. *Human Relations* **13** 95–121.

Montgomery E, Pope C & Rogers J (2015) A feminist narrative study of the maternity care experiences of women who were sexually abused in childhood. *Midwifery* **31** (1) 54–60.

Murray L & Andrews L (2000) *The Social Baby: Understanding babies' communication from birth*. Richmond: CP Publishing.

Parker R (2005) *Torn in Two: The experience of maternal ambivalence*. London: Virago.

Puckering C, Rogers J, Mills M, Cox AD & Mattsson-Graff M (1994) Process and evaluation of a group intervention for mothers with parenting difficulties. *Child Abuse Review* **3** (4) 299–310.

Puckering C, McIntosh E, Hickey A & Longford J (2010) Mellow babies: a group intervention for infants and mothers experiencing postnatal depression. *Counselling Psychology Review* **25** (1) 28–40.

Shapiro V (2009) Reflections on the work of Professor Selma Fraiberg: a pioneer in the field of social work and infant mental health. *Clinial Social Work Journal* **35** 45-55.

Sutton Trust (2014) *Baby Bonds: Parenting, attachment and a secure base for children*. London: Sutton Trust.

Chapter 7: Working with the whole family

Sue Gellhorn

Introduction

Perhaps more than any other area of mental health difficulty, postnatal depression and other maternal mental health difficulties impact significantly on the whole family. Family members are also likely to be key in providing support and help for affected women and in moderating the effect of mental distress on the baby. An NSPCC report (Hogg, 2013) highlights the special context of perinatal mental illness and the need for mental health services to keep the family in mind. This perspective has come to be known as 'Think Family' and there have been a number of service initiatives bridging the needs of parents and children under this heading. This chapter aims to look at the scope for keeping other family members in mind and for informing, involving and intervening with them directly.

Fathers and partners

Fathers and partners, who may or may not be the baby's biological father, are in a position to support a depressed mother but are also at risk of depression themselves. The social and professional support that the parenting couple receive both antenatally and postnatally will have a large influence on their adjustment to parenthood and whether one or both of them become depressed or highly anxious in the perinatal period. It will also affect their resilience as a couple and their capacity to provide support for one another as they care for their new baby (Shrader *et al*, 2009; Underdown, 2012).

Information giving and antenatal education

Almost all online support forums and reports calling for service improvements in perinatal mental health state that parents would have felt better prepared if they had been given more information about mental health issues before the birth (4Children, 2011). Fathers are much less likely to have been given this information than their partners. Both Mind (2014) and the Royal College of Psychiatrists (2015) have excellent information leaflets for partners, friends and relatives.

Antenatal education is undergoing a much needed overhaul and there are some excellent new initiatives building on the research that has indicated where this has been falling short for parents (Department of Health, 2011). Most notable is the Baby Steps perinatal education programme developed by the NSPCC and Warwick University. This is a nine session group programme for mums and dads-to-be which is designed to support parents who may have chaotic lifestyles or who might be considered hard to reach.

The programme is based around relationship building and its key themes reflect the protective factors in the perinatal period. These are:

■ Strengthening parent-infant relationships.

■ Strengthening couple relationships.

■ Building strong support networks.

■ Improving self-confidence as well as levels of mood and worry.

■ Helping parents to understand babies' development.

(Hogg *et al*, 2015)

A key part of Baby Steps is building a strong relationship between parents and their baby, beginning while the baby is still in the womb. Baby Steps works to involve dads and partners in the programme. By supporting fathers in their transition to parenthood it enables them to in turn support their partner. Both parents are encouraged to think and talk about their own feelings and emotions. This new skill in recognising mental states helps them regulate their own emotions and attune to the emotional needs of their babies.

The evaluation of the early programmes has produced a very positive evidence base. Parents who attended:

■ Showed an improvement in the quality of their relationship with their babies.

■ Some had improved satisfaction in their relationship with their partners.

■ Showed increased levels of self-esteem.

■ Had a lower caesarean rate, higher birth weight and fewer premature babies than the general population (Brooks & Coster, 2015).

Supporting partners, buffering babies

The more postnatal depression and perinatal mental health problems are seen in a less medical light and more in psychosocial terms, the more the role of fathers and partners has sparked interest. The Fatherhood Institute (Burgess, 2011) has reviewed the evidence of the father's role in a mother's depression. They identify that research points to a trio of key factors relating to a woman's partner and the likelihood of her developing postnatal depression. They are:

1. Having a poor relationship with her baby's father.

2. The father being unavailable at the time of the baby's birth.

3. The father providing insufficient emotional and practical support (including low participation in infant care).

These are all factors that could potentially be impacted by excellent and inclusive antenatal preparation. This finding is particularly interesting when put together with the finding that 45% of women reported that their husband or partner was the first person they spoke to about mental health difficulties in the perinatal period (Boots Family Trust, 2013).

More positively, there has been awareness of the role of partner support and the potential for fathers to ameliorate the potential negative impact on a baby of its mother's depression. Maternal depression can produce an insensitive response of a mother to her newborn and his needs. This can take the form of relatively 'intrusive or hostile' responses or being 'withdrawn and disengaged'. An example of the former would be a mother who startles or unsettles her baby with an over-loud rattle, failing to pick up his cues that he is finding it too much. An example of a withdrawn and disengaged response would be a mother who barely smiles at her infant over long periods and ignores or responds minimally to her baby's crying. Research has shown that this can cause distress in the baby and impact negatively on their social and emotional development (Murray *et al*, 2010).

A number of studies have found that where mothers were suffering persistent depressive mood, the majority of their infants had established happy relationships with their fathers and had achieved secure attachments to them (Burgess, 2011). Other studies have found that fathers are sometimes able to promote greater responsiveness from the baby's depressed mother and also to minimise her intrusiveness (see Chapter 7). Of course these so-called 'buffering' effects depend on fathers being available and able to get involved in a positive way. There is some evidence that girls are more likely to be protected by father involvement as studies have shown particularly high levels of interaction from fathers with insecure-avoidant girls. These baby girls have developed an insecure attachment to their mothers and have tried to cope, or regulate their emotional state, by avoiding or turning away from contact with their mothers and then benefit a great deal from positive and sensitive involvement from their fathers.

The important learning point is that for fathers to provide this kind of support they need to be well informed about maternal mental health, involved in maternity and health visiting services and respected and supported in their role as a key carer and family member.

Fathers' own depression

The transition to parenthood is a big role shift for fathers as well as mothers. However, the shape of services today means that support from professionals is structured around the needs of women rather than a parenting couple. There is also a lot of encouragement for men to be supportive to their partners. While studies show high levels of anxiety in expectant fathers, professionals, friends and family focus their attention on the mother and baby. In difficult situations, such as miscarriage and the loss of a baby, men may hold back their own feelings of loss and grief in order to support their partner.

The understanding of depression in new fathers is in its infancy. Nevertheless, it has been noted that new fathers show double the rate of depression than the rest of the population of men of the same age. First time fathers are particularly prone to depression. Another group of fathers at greater risk are very young fathers and fathers with very low income. A previous history of depression and a poor relationship with their partner, especially where there has been disagreement about the pregnancy also raises the risk. The Fatherhood Institute recommends that all fathers need education to recognise the signs and symptoms of depression and support to access help in father-friendly, non-stigmatising ways.

Paternal depression is beginning to be recognised as having a negative impact on babies and young children. In families where there is depression in both parents, an unsettled and difficult to soothe baby and issues between the couple, teasing out possible causal relationships becomes a very complex task. What is clear, however, is that where there is depression in both parents the outcomes are even worse for their baby. For example, where both parents are depressed they are least likely to follow good health guidelines, such as putting babies to sleep on their back, breastfeeding and not putting them to bed with a bottle.

Services talking to fathers

The Baby Steps programme and children's centre initiatives of fathers' groups are good examples of services talking to fathers. The report *Building Resilience in Families Under Stress* (Sawyer, 2009) highlights the need for services to target and structure their services towards men. The claim that services often make, that 'We are for everyone, but fathers don't come', does not address the issue adequately. They point out that it is the responsibility of services to market for and target men in more creative and thoughtful ways. Employing designated male staff and offering activities and venues familiar and comfortable to men is a good start.

Sadly, the coalition government did not follow through a proposal for new legislation, made in 2008, regarding an advance in fatherhood policy. This was the proposal for a joint birth registration. These plans for joint birth registration for unmarried fathers was intended as an acknowledgement that engaging with fathers around the births of their babies is a 'golden opportunity moment' for intervention with them. The intention was that this legal requirement would bring much more in terms of a knock-on effect of father's engagement with services and in their children's lives (DWP, 2008). The corollary of this expectation of fathers is that perinatal services must acknowledge and address fathers directly.

Practical steps for involving and supporting fathers

1. Talk to the baby's father antenatally and postnatally (don't just ask him if he has any questions).

2. Build on his strengths – emphasise the positives in his relationship with his baby (Puckering, 2009).

3. Be pro-active in service design – for example, use male-friendly venues and 'techie' approaches to information giving, such as smartphone apps.

4. Enlist the baby's mother to help with engagement of fathers.

5. Make formal referrals of men to male only services.

6. Use male staff to engage fathers and develop male-friendly services.

7. Consider a dads-only antenatal session for men to share pre-birth concerns.

8. Consider referral for couples therapy as an intervention for depression in one or both parents and to protect the baby.

Services for bereaved families and post-adoption

Sometimes there are very serious and sad outcomes for families as a result of perinatal mental ill health.

Perinatal suicide

Despite improving perinatal mental health services across the UK there are sadly a small number of pregnant women and mothers who commit suicide every year. A woman's surviving family need especially sensitive support to cope with their bereavement. Grief after suicide is often complex. Feelings of guilt and anger may be more powerful than in other kinds of bereavement. Support is most likely to fall to GPs and potentially health visitors. The NSPCC (Hogg, 2013) outline what good provision for bereaved families in these circumstances includes:

- Information about how to cope with bereavement and what services there are available.

- The opportunity to discuss issues with a primary care professional, such as a GP.

- The opportunity to discuss issues with obstetric, midwifery services and psychiatric services as appropriate.

- The chance to access one-to-one support or group support for those that need it.

- Outreach and specialist support for those who are particularly vulnerable or traumatised.

If there are older children in the family, the involvement of Child and Adolescent Mental Health Services is likely to be helpful in supporting them in coming to an understanding of what has happened to their family.

Family support post-adoption

Despite common fears among mothers experiencing perinatal mental health difficulties, the removal of a baby from a mother with such problems is rare (see Chapter 7). Where a baby is removed into social services care for this reason it is likely that the family are facing multiple adversities in addition to mental health issues. Mothers who experience the loss of a child in this way need support to help them deal with this outcome. Sadly, therapeutic help for these women is not always available. It is worth noting that for women with severe mental illness, the instigation of care proceedings for their baby appears to increase the risk of suicide. This means that in addition to offers of support, adequate supervision and close communication between health and social care services are especially important.

Babies and other children

Babies and young children in the family where a mother is depressed are usually very sensitive to their mother's moods. But they themselves are at the stage of development where they need help from adult carers to manage their own experiences and feelings. For a baby it can be frightening and distressing to get no response or no smile back from their mother. This is because the baby's own sense of self is dependent on this sort of interpersonal feedback. This observation about babies has been used in studies of infant attachment, where it is referred to as the 'still face' paradigm (Tronick *et al*, 1978).

Babies are very different, come into the world with different temperaments and may respond and attempt to 'cope' with a depressed mother in different ways. It is important for professionals to understand that reports of 'easy' and 'good' babies may hide difficulties for the baby that need picking up on and attending to, as much as concerns about so-called 'difficult' or 'fussy' babies.

Undemanding babies

Undemanding babies may sleep a lot at night and in the day. Depressed mothers may feel relieved that their baby is making so few demands on them but their baby will be missing out on opportunities for bonding with their mother and some of the day-to-day stimulation and involvement in family life that facilitates their development at this very early stage.

'Good' babies

So-called 'good' babies find a way of being which is easy to please, responsive and rewarding for the adults around them. These babies may well grow up into children who feel responsible for looking after their mother – sometimes referred to as a 'parental child'. But this means they have missed out on adult help, or 'containment' (see Chapter 4) to help them recognise and regulate their own emotional states.

'Demanding' babies

These babies may cry for long periods and give their mother the impression that they can never be satisfied or that nothing is quite right for them. This is challenging for any new mother but particularly for a mother who is depressed.

All these situations can benefit from a thoughtful professional or third party who is able to notice and think about the baby's needs from more neutral ground. Chapter 4 has already considered some of the approaches that work explicitly with mother-infant interaction and the mother's capacity to hold her baby and his or her emotional state in mind. It is encouraging to note that early indications are that interventions working with mother-infant interactions can alleviate symptoms of maternal depression even when these are not targeted per se (Barlow *et al*, 2008).

The mother's own mother and extended family

Many mothers experiencing postnatal depression or other maternal mental health difficulties are much supported by their own mother or mother-in-law. However this potentially beneficial relationship is also often fraught with tension, distress and disappointment. This may be difficulty with a withdrawn or unavailable mother figure and the converse; the intrusive, controlling mother. Just as infants struggle with these sorts of mothering, so do new mothers struggle with their relationship with their mother or mother-in-law.

Some women will feel a lack of interest and support from their own mother which stirs up angry resentment and painful re-evaluations of their own childhood experiences. Of course, some women may have lost their mother in childhood, in adulthood or very close to the time of their giving birth, and these new mothers will have the task of grieving again for their mothers just at a time when they understand firsthand what being a mother means.

Other women will feel intruded upon and suffocated by an excess of 'help' and advice from their mother, and feel as if she is taking over too much and even competing for the role of primary carer for the newborn. This sort of experience has parallels with the baby who feels that he or she can never explore a new toy or experience because the mother is showing them how it is done before any exploration can take place.

Relationships with mothers-in-law can be similarly supportive and valuable or fraught and conflicted. Mothers can feel that they are unable to set boundaries on their mother-in-law's involvement and negotiate with their partners on whose job it is to be assertive around the new territory. In some cultures this is particularly tough as new mothers may be expected to live in the household of their in-laws and even look after the wider family as well as their newborn (CPHVA, 2003).

Conclusion

This chapter has been a reminder that when we treat and support a new mother for depression and anxiety we also need to keep in mind that we are treating a whole family. The new mother is presenting her difficulties in the context of all her family relationships: her relationship with her newborn, with her other children, if she has any (and previous stillbirths and miscarriages), her husband or partner, her own parents and in-laws and her friends and extended social network. This means that her symptoms need to be understood in the context of all her relationships and her history of being parented. This perspective helps service providers to be oriented to helping her:

- ask for and accept offers of help and support

- let her partner in to find his own unique way of parenting and relating to his baby

- work on communication with and the needs and expectations of others

- manage her feelings about her own mother as she learns to mother her baby

- set boundaries and manage the shifting nature of new family roles and relationships.

References

4Children (2011) *Suffering in Silence: 70,000 reasons why help with postnatal depression has to be better* [online]. Available at: www.4children.org.uk/Resources/Detail/Suffering-in-Silence (accessed April 2016).

Barlow J, Schrader McMillan A, Smith A, Ghate D & Barnes J (2008) *Health-led Parenting Interventions in Pregnancy and the Early Years* [online]. Research Report DCSF-RWO70. London: Department of Children, Schools and Families. Available at: http://dera.ioe.ac.uk/id/eprint/8573 (accessed April 2016).

Boots Family Trust (2013) *Perinatal Mental Health: Experiences of women and health professionals* [online]. Available at: http://www.bftalliance.co.uk/the-report/ (accessed April 2016).

Brooks H & Coster D (2015) *Evaluation of the Baby Steps Programme: Pre- and post-measures study* [online]. NSPCC, Impact and Evidence Series. Available at: http://www.nspcc.org.uk/globalassets/documents/research-reports/baby-steps-evaluation-pre-post-measures-study.pdf (accessed January 2016).

Burgess A (2011) *Father's Roles in Perinatal Mental Health: Causes, interactions and effects* [online]. Fatherhood Institute, New Digest 53, NCT. Available at: http://www.academia.edu/3523803/Fathers_roles_in_perinatal_mental_health (accessed April 2016).

CPHVA (2003) *Understanding our Emotional Health Needs: What helps? Perspectives from black and ethnic minority communities*. CPHVA Conference Proceedings, Sheffield, 2003.

Department of Health (2011) *Preparation for Birth and Beyond: A resource pack for leaders of community groups and activities* [online]. Available at: https://www.gov.uk/government/publications/preparation-for-birth-and-beyond-a-resource-pack-for-leaders-of-community-groups-and-activities (accessed April 2016).

Department for Work and Pensions (2008) *Joint Birth Registration: Recording responsibility* [online]. Available at: https://www.gov.uk/government/uploads/system/uploads/attachment_data/file/243115/7293.pdf (accessed April 2016).

Hogg S (2013) *Prevention in Mind. All Babies Count: Spotlight on perinatal mental health* [online]. NSPCC. Available at: http://everyonesbusiness.org.uk/wp-content/uploads/2014/06/NSPCC-Spotlight-report-on-Perinatal-Mental-Health.pdf (accessed April 2016).

Hogg S, Coster D & Brooks H (2015) *Baby Steps: Evidence from a relationships-based perinatal education programme* [online]. NSPCC. Available at: www.aimh.org.uk/pdf/news/20150219195927.pdf (accessed April 2016).

Mind (2014) *Understanding Postnatal Depression* [online]. Available at: http://www.mind.org.uk/media/46890/understanding_postnatal_depression_2013.pdf (accessed April 2016).

Murray l, Halligan S & Cooper P (2010) Effects of postnatal depression on mother-infant interactions and child development. In: JG Bremner and TD Wachs (Eds) *Handbook of Infant Development, Vol.2* (2nd edition). Oxford: Wiley Blackwell.

Puckering C (2009) Mellow Babies: Mellow Parenting with parents of infants. In: Barlow J and Svanberg PO (Eds) *Keeping the Baby in Mind* (pp155-163). London: Routledge.

Royal College of Psychiatrists (2015) *Postnatal Depression* [online]. Partners in Care Campaign. Available at: http://www.rcpsych.ac.uk/healthadvice/partnersincarecampaign/postnataldepression.aspx (accessed April 2016).

Sawyer E (2009) *Building Resilience in Families Under Stress: Supporting families affected by parental substance misuse and/or mental health problems*. London: National Children's Bureau Enterprises Ltd.

Schrader McMillan A, Barlow J & Redshaw M (2009) *Birth and Beyond: A review of the evidence about antenatal education* [online]. University of Warwick/University of Oxford

Tronick E, Als H, Adamson L, Wise S & Brazelton TB (1978) The infant's response to entrapment between contradictory messages in face-to-face interaction. *Journal of the American Academy of Child Psychiatry* **17** 1–3.

Underdown A (2012) *Baby Steps: A perinatal programme*. London: NSPCC.

Understanding Childhood (2014) *Postnatal Depression: A problem for the whole family* [online] Available at: http://www.understandingchildhood.net/posts/post-natal-depression-a-problem-for-all-the-family/ (accessed April 2016).

Chapter 8: Supporting mothers in complex family contexts

Sue Gellhorn

As we have already seen in earlier chapters, a baby's early path in the world is influenced by a story that begins well before his birth. It is shaped by his parents' expectations and plans, their relationship, their backgrounds and well-being, and the social and political circumstances they find themselves in as they approach parenthood. This chapter is about some of the complex family contexts into which babies in the UK are currently born.

Migrants, asylum seekers and refugees

Research has shown that health professionals find it easier to provide services to UK-born mothers from minority ethnic groups than to migrant mothers who may be new to the health system as well as the language and culture of the UK (Puthussery *et al*, 2008). Patterns of migration to the UK are changing all the time. In 2011, Polish women were the most numerous group of non-UK-born mothers giving birth in the UK. It is helpful to be clear about definitions in this discussion, as terms are sometimes used interchangeably and without recognition of their legal and psychological implications for service delivery.

Migrants

Migrants are a very heterogeneous group and include new migrants, who may have been in the UK for a very short period of time, and 'long-term migrants', who have been living in the UK or their country of destination for at least a year. Migrants include economic migrants, asylum seekers, refugees, as well as people coming to the UK with a visa for study, as tourists, for work or for marriage. The refugee council gives useful information about the terminology relating to asylum seekers and refugees in the UK (www.refugeecouncil.org.uk).

- An asylum seeker is someone who has made a formal application to the Home Office for temporary protection, asylum or humanitarian protection.

- A refugee is someone who has been granted discretionary leave, asylum or protection because they are at risk of persecution if they return to their home country.

- A failed asylum seeker has had their application refused but under the appeal system they may still be formally seeking asylum.

The 2011 triennial report of maternal deaths in the UK (Oates & Cantwell, 2011) reported that newly arrived migrants, refugees and asylum-seeking women are over-represented in the figures for maternal death from domestic abuse or other causes. They suggest that this is for a complex mix of reasons. The vulnerability of these women was highlighted in the report by some particularly sad cases. Two such cases involved the murder by family members of brides who had recently arrived in the UK, both of whom were young Asian women who did not speak English; a further two died through suicide or accidental death in suspicious circumstances. They noted common features of poor treatment of these women by their new families and collusion within the family as factors in these deaths. The centre recommends that health professionals monitor this group of often very young women closely.

Case example: Dirribe

Dirribe is a young Sudanese woman who was trafficked into west London in her late teens. She worked in domestic service where she was badly treated by her 'employer'. Eventually she ran away and was helped by the police to access support from a voluntary sector project for trafficked women and girls. In a hostel for homeless young people she had a brief relationship with a teenage refugee and became pregnant with her first child. As she approached motherhood alone and with little English she was also seeking asylum through the formal channels. She faced multiple challenges accessing services because of her age, legal status, homelessness and poverty. In time, however, she was very well supported through a trusting relationship with her family nurse and the counsellor in a local GP surgery who was able to continue seeing her despite her numerous moves in and out of temporary accommodation. She never spoke in detail about her past experiences but valued the professional help and 'mothering' of those working with her as she began to enjoy being a mother to her baby daughter and meeting other young mothers at a nearby children's centre.

Maternity Action, a voluntary sector organisation campaigning for better maternity care for all groups of women, point to the negative impact of UK Border Agency (UKBA) dispersal policies, despite the new guidance for protected periods for pregnant women and new mothers introduced in 2012. Their report shows the impact of dispersal and relocation on women's health and experiences of pregnancy, birth and becoming a new mother (Maternity Action, 2013).

These experiences include women:

- being moved away from midwives, GPs and special support that they trust and understand, and suffering serious mental health problems before and after birth

- being separated from their family and social network and, in some instances, the father of their baby and finding themselves in an unfamiliar city

- being moved multiple times during pregnancy, often to crowded and dirty accommodation where they feel unsafe and unable to care for their babies

- giving birth alone, without a birth partner

- having no cash for basic amenities for their baby or for transport.

There are some indications that migrant women miss out on mental health assessments, perhaps as professionals attempt to deal with missing antenatal checks and housing and benefit issues (see Chapter 3). Much of the work done to detect maternal mental health difficulties is dependent on women self-reporting symptoms to practitioners. There are, of course, often language barriers, but there are also many cultural issues around differing perceptions of psychological difficulties. Latif (2014) identifies some of these as:

- women reporting to practitioners – 'We never talk about these things'

- women presenting with somatic concerns, for example, aches and pains, pressure in the head, 'hot' feelings and so on

- fear of stigmatisation and being shunned by the community.

Being aware of the above issues, failings and challenges will help practitioners to be as sensitive and reflective in their own practice as possible. Some more practical steps for service providers to incorporate in attempting to meet this area of need are:

- Make use of same-language workers, such as link workers, assistant psychologists and family support workers.

- Always use professional interpreters (not family members, including children).

- Listen and ask about a woman's experiences and culture rather than relying on limited bits of cultural knowledge.

- Start with the needs of the community (for example, courses may be more popular than 'therapy' groups).

- Remember that even within a particular culture, including your own, there is huge variation.

(Marks *et al*, 2009)

Case example: Ardiana

Ardiana had had a very difficult birth with her second child. She suffered a severe postpartum haemorrhage and was in intensive care for five days. Soon after her daughter's birth, she heard of her sister's death back at home in Kosovo. She felt very cut-off from her family of origin and had no real opportunity to grieve for her sister. Once physically recovered and back at home with her new baby and older child she felt she was no longer a 'strong' mother to her new baby and felt inadequate and unable to care for her properly. She felt jumpy and over-anxious and found it difficult to take the children out to the shops. She was tired all the time and felt ashamed of what she saw as weakness, having previously seen herself as strong and energetic.

She was troubled by memories from her childhood of traumatic family separations during the war in Kosovo and was worried about family members still living there. Her husband was supportive but she often called him at work to come home and help her with the children. She spoke very little English and did not feel comfortable leaving the children with a child-minder, but because she felt desperate she took up her health visitor's suggestion that she make an appointment with a psychologist specialising in perinatal difficulties. With the help of an interpreter, who made efforts to be available for each session, and with her two small children with her in the sessions, Ardiana was able to put her memories, fears and anxieties into words and begin to regain her previous confidence and vitality.

There are examples of good practice across the UK that may be applicable in your local services (NICE, 2012). For instance, the 'Refugee specialist' midwife working in Manchester is an example of service development tailored to emerging population need.

The Barking and Dagenham PCT information resource 'The Maternity Wheel' (see Figure 8.1) is an example of excellent bottom-up service development, involving migrant women, young people and ethnic minority communities. In collaboration with the Polyanna project, they developed an attractive, user-friendly information 'wheel' to encourage so-called hard-to-reach groups to find their way to the help they need.

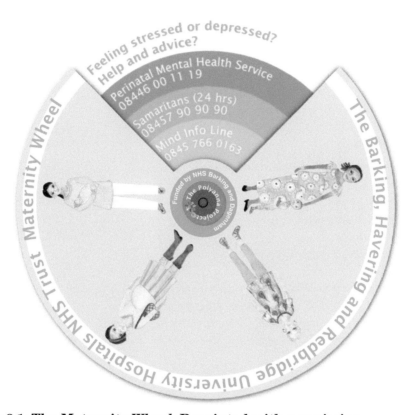

Figure 8.1: The Maternity Wheel. Reprinted with permission from Homeyard C, Gaudion A and Cutts H. The Polyanna Project. Available from: http://www.thepolyannaproject.org.uk/documents/ BHRUTreport12-3-10.pdf (accessed April 2016)

Liz McDonald, perinatal psychiatrist, describes how providing services for migrant women with a range of backgrounds can work:

'We acknowledge that many women may be at different stages along the spectrum of acculturation or they may feel alienated both within the wider community and within the community that develops in the unit. Asylum seekers and refugees are not a homogeneous group and are different to the settled refugee population. Their health problems are often related to their country of origin and therefore we take particular care to ensure that their physical health needs are attended to.'
(Liz McDonald, perinatal psychiatrist quoted in Edge, 2011)

Women living with domestic violence

There will be a proportion of women on any midwife or health visitor's caseload, or attending a six-week postnatal check with a GP, or buying nappies in the supermarket, who will be subject to violence or abuse at home. By the nature of their role, midwives and health visitors are often the first to become aware of domestic violence within a family. This presents both an opportunity and a challenge to these healthcare providers. Junior health staff are often the first to be confided in and need support from experienced professionals to manage some of the troubling stories they are told (Marks *et al*, 2009).

Definitions

Domestic violence and abuse is defined as:

'Any incident, or pattern of incidents of controlling, coercive or threatening behaviour, violence or abuse (psychological, physical, sexual, financial or emotional) between those aged 16 or over who are or have been intimate partners or family members, regardless of gender or sexuality.

Controlling behaviour is acting in a way that is designed to make a person subordinate and/or dependent by isolating them from sources of support, exploiting their resources and capacities for personal gain, depriving them of the means needed for independence, resistance and escape, and regulating their everyday behaviour.

Coercive behaviour is an act or pattern of acts of assault, threats, humiliation and intimidation or other abuse that is used to harm, punish or frighten the victim.'
(Department of Health, 2013)

Harsh realities for this group of child-bearing women

- In the 2006–08 CMACE triennial report, 34 of the women who had died from any cause had features of domestic abuse in their case.

- Assessing all deaths in the above report, 17 mothers were identified who had reported childhood sexual abuse by a relative.

- Pregnancy and new motherhood offer no protection from abuse – in fact, some abuse begins or is exacerbated during pregnancy.

- Multiple social adversity increases the likelihood of perinatal victimisation by an abuser.

Department of Health (2013) guidance for health visitors identifies a so-called 'toxic trio' of domestic violence, mental ill-health and substance misuse. These three factors are viewed as indicators of increased risk of harm to children and young people who are living in such families. Where all three factors are present in families, the risks to babies and children are very great.

Lutz (2005) has described the very bleak continuity of past and present violence for women in her qualitative study of 12 survivors of domestic violence. These women reported many types of violence at different points in their lives. They had often experienced childhood physical, emotional and sexual abuse, neglect, parental partner violence and substance abuse, current domestic violence, sexual assault, and community violence. For these women, intimate partner violence during childbearing was part of a continuum of abusive experiences across the narrative of their lives.

Antenatal care for women suffering abuse

Women experiencing domestic abuse may have particular difficulties accessing antenatal care services. The perpetrator of their abuse may try to prevent them from getting to appointments. The woman herself may be fearful that disclosure of abuse may worsen her situation and may be worried about the reaction of health professionals if she does disclose abuse. Allowing for flexibility over the frequency and length of appointments for vulnerable groups of women increases the likelihood that their circumstances will become known and they may then be able to access help at some stage.

Both the NICE guidelines on pregnancy and complex social factors (2012) and the CMACE report (Oates & Cantwell, 2011) recommend health practitioners asking about domestic violence at repeated health contacts during the maternity journey. The evidence is that women do not disclose at the first enquiry. Statistics show that on average women will experience 35 assaults before going to the police. Professionals must also guard against presumptions about the sort of women seen as likely victims. CMACE points out that domestic abuse occurs across all social classes and ethnic groups and that health professionals are victims of abuse too.

Case example: Iryna

Iryna had come to London from the Ukraine to study accountancy. While studying, she became pregnant by her boyfriend who worked in the city. During pregnancy she noticed a change in the way he treated her and she became worried about his weekend 'partying', which involved heavy use of recreational drugs. Feeling unsupported and unable to continue work and her studies, she became depressed. After the baby was born a health visitor referred the family to social services because of concern about the baby's father's drug use. At the social services assessment Iryna's boyfriend dominated the discussion and reported that he was no longer using drugs and that Iryna was over-anxious and 'unstable' because of her postnatal depression. After visiting her own family for support, Iryna was re-referred to an IAPT (Improving Access to Psychological Therapies) psychologist, who helped her think about how her boyfriend had been treating her and how this impacted on her relationship with her baby. As she began to feel more positive about herself and the kind of home life she wanted for her baby, she finally felt strong enough to make the decision that it would be better to raise her daughter as a single mother.

Asking about domestic violence

The Department of Health (2013) professional guidance on domestic violence and abuse outlines the knowledge base and practical considerations required to ask women if they are suffering abuse or violence at home in an effective manner. Below are the steps they outline for asking somebody about domestic violence.

Ensure it is safe to ask

Consider the environment:

■ Is it conducive to ask?

■ Is it safe to ask?

■ Never ask in the presence of another family member, friend, or child over the age of two years.

Create the opportunity to ask the question. Use an appropriate professional interpreter (never a family member).

Ask

Frame the topic first then ask a direct question. Examples:

Framing: *'As violence in the home is so common we now ask contacts about it routinely.'*

Direct Question: *'Are you in a relationship with someone who hurts or threatens you?'*
'Did someone cause these injuries to you?'

Validate

Validate what's happening to the individual and send important messages to the contact:

'You are not alone.'

'You are not to blame for what is happening to you.'

'You do not deserve to be treated in this way.'

Assess

Assess contact's safety:

'Is your partner here with you?'

'Where are the children?'

'Do you have any immediate concerns?'

'Do you have a place of safety?'

Action

Be aware of your local domestic violence agency, how to contact a local independent domestic violence advisor (IDVA), offer leaflet and suggest referral. Action any local safeguarding procedures.

Document

Consider safety and confidentiality when recording information in patient notes. Medical records can be used by survivors in future criminal justice proceedings. (Department of Health, 2013)

It is important to recognise that it is the health professional's role to validate and support women but not to pass comment or encourage a woman to leave her partner.

Child protection and safeguarding

Child protection and safeguarding concerns are particularly pertinent for families where domestic abuse is taking place or is suspected. The work may involve:

- making an assessment of the risk to the babies and children in the household

- explaining the limits of confidentiality and safeguarding responsibilities

- giving information about the impact of domestic violence on children

- collaborating with the named nurse for Safeguarding Children and Domestic Violence Lead

- making a referral to the Multi Agency Risk Assessment Committee (MARAC)

■ keeping detailed electronic records of any injuries and a woman's reports – but never in hand-held maternity records or the Personal Child Health Record (PCHR or 'red book').

(Dennis, 2014)

Supporting homeless mothers and babies

Researchers and politicians refer to and report on homeless families, but homeless babies are rarely discussed. This was brought home by a recent report by the NSPCC (Hogg, 2013), which discovered that while homeless families with children are recorded, there is no record kept of the numbers of babies in the UK that are statutorily homeless. Homelessness means lacking a place to live that is supportive, affordable, decent and secure. The NSPCC estimates that around 15,000 under-two-year-olds are homeless. Babies that are born into homeless families or become homeless as infants are far less likely to have a healthy and safe start in life. Homelessness compromises the following areas of babies' lives:

■ Healthy development in utero.

■ Healthy early relationship with a sensitive and responsive caregiver.

■ Effective care and support for their caregivers.

■ A safe and stimulating environment.

Homeless families are often referred to as 'hard to reach' by service providers, but unstable housing and frequent moves create multiple obstacles for parents simply to achieve the basics of everyday living. In addition, homeless parents often have their own history of adversity and are likely to have suffered, or be suffering from mental health problems or domestic violence. Frequent moves between hostels, bed and breakfast and short term housing mean that the babies' parent/s – and often a single mother – will be upset, stressed and exhausted, and will not feel positive about the future.

As affordable and social housing are currently in short supply, homeless families can feel under pressure to prove their status as homeless and compete for scarce resources. This pressure challenges the emotional resources of the mother to provide sensitive and responsive care for her baby. In areas where there are specialist health services, midwives and health visitors (for example, the Sheffield Homeless and Traveller Health Team) it is more feasible to offer a joined-up service that can meet the real needs of babies in homeless families. The Family Nurse Partnership also supports many young homeless families by virtue of the overlap of their young, vulnerable target group and homelessness (see the case example of Dirribe).

Sadly, the NSPCC report a review of 40 serious case reviews (Hogg, 2015), which revealed that 45% of these families were highly mobile and living in poor conditions. It is likely that this figure represents significant unmet need for the babies living in these families.

Motherhood after perinatal loss, assisted conception and prematurity

Any new mother faces the psychological challenge of forming a maternal identity alongside the physical gestation process. For women becoming mothers after perinatal loss, assisted conception and prematurity, this process becomes more complicated. Conception and delivery of a live baby do not erase the months or years of failure and loss associated with infertility. There have been attempts to delineate the relationship between mothers conceiving by assisted reproductive technology (ART), such as in vitro fertilisation (IVF), and postnatal depression. However, any correlation is most likely confounded by the older maternal age and prior losses of women conceiving by these means. Similarly, most of the 'high-risk' physical status of pregnancies following ART is associated with so-called 'advanced' maternal age and the conception of multiple embryos.

In all of the circumstances above there is a component of grief in the journey to conception and birth. Mothers may have suffered multiple miscarriages, endured repeated rounds of IVF treatment, or had a prior stillbirth or cot death. In another situation of vulnerability, prematurity brings a bewildering state of motherhood in limbo, where women report being uncertain whether they themselves or the neonatal nursing staff have 'parental' authority over the baby. Any coincidence of grief and pregnancy represents a real psychological challenge, as a life lost must be grieved for alongside the celebration and nurturing of a new life. Raphael-Leff (2009) identifies the heightened emotional investment in such babies and the way this can interact with a mother's inner feelings of confidence or anxiety. She describes the tussle between positive and negative feelings, such as:

hope ----- distrust
elation ----- detachment
idealisation ----- negativity

Midwives and staff working in special care baby units will encounter this to-ing and fro-ing of parental outlook on a daily basis.

References

Dennis T (2014) *Working with Domestic Violence and Abuse: Good practice points for health visitors: Working with minority groups.* London: Institute of Health Visiting.

Department of Health (2013) *Domestic Violence and Abuse – Professional Guidance No.5.* London: DH. Available at: https://www.gov.uk/government/uploads/system/uploads/attachment_data/file/211018/9576-TSO-Health_Visiting_Domestic_Violence_A3_Posters_WEB.pdf (accessed April 2016).

Edge D (2011) *National Perinatal Mental Health Project Report: Perinatal mental health of black and minority ethnic women: A review of current provision in England, Scotland and Wales.* London: National Mental Health Development Unit.

Hogg S (2015) *An Unstable Start: All babies count: Spotlight on homelessness.* London: NSPCC and Anna Freud Centre.

Latif Z (2014) *The Maternal Mental Health of Migrant Women: Better health briefing paper 31.* London: Race Equality Foundation.

Lutz KF (2005) Abuse experiences, perceptions, and associated decisions during the childbearing cycle. *Western Journal of Nursing Research* **27** (7) 802–824.

Marks L, Hadley S, Reay A, Gelman T & Mckay A (2009) Working with parents from black and minority ethnic backgrounds in Children's Centres. In: J Barlow and PO Svanberg (Eds) *Keeping the Baby in Mind* (pp128–138). London: Routledge.

Maternity Action (2013) *When Maternity Doesn't Matter: Dispersing pregnant women seeking asylum* [online]. Available at: www.refugeecouncil.org.uk/maternity (accessed April 2016).

NICE (2012) *Pregnancy and Complex Social Factors: A model for service provision for pregnant women with complex social factors* (NICE Clinical Guideline 110). London: NICE.

Oates M & Cantwell R (2011) Deaths from psychiatric causes. In: Centre for Maternal and Child Enquiries (CMACE) Saving Mothers' Lives: Reviewing Maternal Deaths To Make Motherhood Safer: 2006-08. *BJOG* **118** (S1) 1–203.

Puthussery S, Twamley K, Harding S, Mirsky J, Baron M & Macfarlane A (2008) 'They're more like ordinary stroppy British women': attitudes and expectations of maternity care professionals to UK-born ethnic minority women. *Journal of Health Service Research and Policy* **13** (4) 195–201.

Raphael-Leff J (2009) *Psychological Processes of Childbearing* (4th edition). London: Anna Freud Centre.

Chapter 9: Severe perinatal mental health difficulties

Agnieszka Klimowicz and Elizabeth Best

Midwives and health visitors will be familiar with situations in which a pregnant woman or a mother who has given birth suffers from depression or increased anxiety. The authors of this chapter, who work in a specialist perinatal mental health service and have had many conversations with midwives and health visitors over the years, would like to share information regarding mental health difficulties that occur less frequently, but which usually create more worries among healthcare and social care professionals. It is our assumption that better understanding in this respect will be helpful in providing well timed, sensitive and appropriate responses from the services.

The importance of severe mental health difficulties around the time of delivery was evidenced in Kendell *et al*'s (1987) study *Epidemiology of Puerperal Psychoses*. The authors concluded that 'the "relative risk" of admission to a psychiatric hospital with a psychotic illness was extremely high in the first 30 days after childbirth'. It is now accepted that the presence of certain risk factors might translate into a deterioration of mental state during and after pregnancy. We would like to describe those factors, as well as outlining what healthcare services can do to help prevent and treat severe mental health problems. One of the functions of a specialist perinatal mental health service is to offer help to midwives and health visitors in detecting women who are vulnerable to relapse of severe mental illness and puerperal psychosis, and to refer them on.

Overview of the major disorders

Severe mental illness (SMI), as defined by the National Institute for Care and Health Excellence (NICE), includes severe and incapacitating depression, psychosis, schizophrenia, bipolar affective disorder, schizoaffective disorder and postpartum psychosis.

To describe SMI, we will use the tenth revision of the International Classification of Mental and Behavioural Disorders (ICD-10) (WHO, 1992). This classification is widely used in Europe.

Contrary to many other fields in medicine, there are no laboratory investigations confirming psychiatric diagnoses, although they are commonly used to differentiate functional problems from organic ones (i.e. those resulting from infection, pain, intoxication or drug overdose, and other physical problems). As a result, ICD-10 uses the term 'disorder' rather than 'disease'.

According to ICD-10 disorder implies 'the existence of a clinically recognizable set of symptoms or behaviour associated in most cases with distress and with interference with personal functions', and is not an exact term. Furthermore, psychiatrists are encouraged to diagnose as many disorders as required to explain the clinical presentation, and it is therefore not unusual for a person to be diagnosed with two or more disorders.

The medical term disease is used when the underlying aetiology is known. In cases of psychiatric problems, the causality is very frequently considered multifactorial, and the factors can be divided into:

- predisposing (e.g. genetic)
- precipitating (e.g. hormonal changes after delivery)
- perpetuating (e.g. availability of the suitable treatment, individual's compliance).

These can be divided further into bio-psycho-social subcategories. Careful history taking allows for identification of those factors. In return, it helps to inform care plans offering the best support and the interventions to reduce the impact of these factors on the individual's mental state, and thus promotes recovery. The involvement of family members in care plans should be organised whenever possible, and the well-being of children should be considered at every professional contact.

Depression versus transiently depressed mood (baby blues)

The most common mental health problem occurring during pregnancy and following birth is, as at any other time, depression (about 10–15%). It is estimated that about one-third to half of women with depression in pregnancy and after delivery suffer from its severe form, which requires specialist help, and treatment with medication is usually recommended.

Depression is usually an episodic condition, however, it can also be chronic. As in many other psychiatric problems, it is important to sensitively establish factors that might maintain the depression. These could include a woman's psychosocial situation (e.g. domestic violence, lack of support, economic pressures), vulnerability associated with personality (e.g. learned helplessness), undiagnosed physical health problems (e.g. thyroid problems), substance misuse, or suboptimal treatment.

It is important to differentiate between a depressive episode and transient and mild symptoms, called 'baby blues', which occur in about 50–80% of women within the first few days after delivery. The former is usually diagnosed when symptoms last for longer than 14 days, and will not resolve with a good night's sleep and support from loved ones. However, a new onset depressive episode starting around the time of delivery, with severe symptoms (and severely impairing everyday functioning) requires specialist psychiatric attention without delay.

The main symptoms of depression include:

- depressed mood
- loss of interest and enjoyment
- reduced energy
- tiredness
- diminished activity.

Other symptoms can include:

- reduced concentration and attention
- reduced self-esteem and self-confidence
- ideas of guilt and unworthiness (these might involve thinking about being a 'bad mother')
- pessimistic views of the future
- ideas or acts of self-harm or suicide
- disturbed sleep
- diminished appetite.

For the diagnosis of severe depression, at least three main symptoms and four other symptoms should be present. Women who have a history of depression before pregnancy are at increased risk of its reoccurrence after delivery (30-40%), particularly if they have suffered a previous depression postnatally (50%). However, the best predictor of postnatal depression is a depression during pregnancy. It is therefore important to support and treat women when the problem is identified.

Women with severe depression might have difficulty attending to complex tasks after delivery, may give up breastfeeding, and may suffer a loss of joy and warm feelings towards their baby. This, together with the presence of guilty feelings, may lead them to feel that they are not good mothers and to criticise themselves. These problems usually disappear with treatment (both pharmacological and psychosocial), when the source of the problem is anhedonia resulting from depression. If depression occurs in the context of maternal attachment insecurity, pharmacological intervention alone is unlikely to improve the emerging problem in the mother-infant relationship.

In some circumstances, particularly when a woman is untreated and suffers suicidal thoughts, there might be a risk to both the mother and the baby. Women might be reluctant to admit to the scope of their depressive thinking, worried that their baby will be taken away, and thus not receive treatment at all until they are very unwell or someone around them is very concerned. As one of the authors' patients said: 'I will not tell you, doctor, what I think, as you will refer me to social services'. This statement, interpreted by the patient's psychiatrist as her wish to open up, alongside her uncertainty as to its benefits, was followed by a more in-depth conversation, with an explanation regarding social services' role. An increased level of support and adjustment of medication was arranged as a result. The referral to social services was not required at this stage.

Women with severe depression might also suffer from psychotic symptoms (see p.120: 'Psychosis') or might suffer from accompanying anxiety symptoms. They might be preoccupied with irrational worries or have obsessive thoughts and compulsive behaviours.

Hypomanic and manic episode versus transiently elated mood (baby pinks)

About 15% of women experience transiently elated mood in the first days after delivery. In its mild form, mood is excellent with lots of positive feelings. This is not a mental health problem per se, and the phenomenon is known as 'baby pinks'. However, when it persists for more than a few days, and is associated with inability to fall asleep or reduced need to sleep, lack of tiredness, talkativeness that is out of character, grandiose ideas, and/or irresponsible behaviour, it may indicate that a woman is suffering from a hypomanic episode. This will require pharmacological treatment, as it can progress to a more ominous manic episode, needing management in hospital owing to almost complete disruption of usual activity, and in its most severe form can lead to losing touch with reality due to psychotic symptoms (puerperal psychosis).

Bipolar affective disorder

Particularly vulnerable to severe mood changes (both severe depression and hypomanic and manic episodes, with or without psychotic symptoms) are women with an established diagnosis of bipolar affective disorder (BPAD), and the risk of puerperal psychosis is estimated in this group to be about 50%. In comparison, the risk of puerperal psychosis after any delivery is one to two per 1,000 (0.1-0.2%). A puerperal, first ever hypomanic or manic episode, even without psychotic symptoms, might also be an indicator of BPAD.

For BPAD to be diagnosed, at least two episodes of mood disturbance must occur, in which 'the patient's mood and activity levels are significantly disturbed' (ICD-10), and at least one of them will be associated with elated mood (hypomanic, manic or mixed affective episode). BPAD affects about one per cent of the general population. It usually starts in late adolescence or early adulthood. Recovery is usually complete between the episodes.

Puerperal psychosis

This is an umbrella term, usually reserved for very severe forms of mood disorder with psychotic symptoms starting typically (estimated in 95% of cases) in the first two weeks after delivery. It may be an indicator of BPAD, or schizoaffective disorder, but the minority of women with puerperal psychosis (PP) will be later diagnosed with, or might already have an established diagnosis of, schizophrenia. There are also women who suffer from PP who have not experienced episodes of mood disorder prior to pregnancy. It is presently thought that the main biological factor triggering PP is associated with sensitivity to hormonal changes following delivery. However, other factors, such as being a new mother or delivering by caesarean section, seem to increase the risk of PP.

A woman with PP will usually require hospitalisation. Whenever possible this should be at a psychiatric mother and baby unit in order to prevent separation and thus further complications, including bonding problems. Prompt pharmacological treatment and psychosocial interventions alongside an appropriate level of care will in most cases be sufficient to achieve recovery. The involvement of family members in planning the post discharge care and support, whenever possible, is vital.

Puerperal psychosis should be treated as a psychiatric emergency, and is considered a high risk of harm to the mother and the baby.

In women with an established diagnosis of SMI, or history of SMI (including history of PP), the risk of PP might be reduced by prophylactic use of mood stabiliser or mood stabilising antipsychotics in pregnancy (or towards the end of pregnancy/early after delivery). The decision should be made by a psychiatrist (whenever possible by a perinatal psychiatrist) with the woman, and must be acceptable to her.

Psychosis

This is a general term describing clinical conditions in which the disturbance of thinking and perception amounts to various degrees of loss of contact with reality. The person might suffer delusions (false beliefs that are not subject to reason and/ or contradictory evidence, and cannot be explained by a person's usual cultural and religious concepts), and/or hallucinations (perceptual abnormalities, when a person can see, hear, smell, taste or feel something that is not there, and has no or very limited ability to distinguish those experiences from real perceptions – see the case example of Sasha). Both delusions and hallucinations can be treated with antipsychotic medications.

Psychotic symptoms characterise conditions such as schizophrenia (according to ICD-10: if psychotic symptoms last for longer than one month) or schizoaffective disorder (in which they occur alongside severe mood disturbance). Schizophrenia, similarly to BPAD, affects about one per cent of the population, and it usually starts in late adolescence or early adulthood.

Hallucinations and delusions in schizophrenia are frequently referred to as 'positive' symptoms (so called to acknowledge that the experience is excessive). Disturbance of thought process also belongs to this group.

Cognitive impairment and 'negative' symptoms of schizophrenia (such as marked apathy, poverty of speech, blunted affect, social withdrawal, lowering of social performance) are less amenable to pharmacological treatment and more likely to interfere with everyday functioning in the longer term. The person's insight regarding their mental illness might influence their willingness to receive treatment and contribute to the prevention (or not) of future psychotic episodes. Therefore, this group of symptoms might have a longer-term impact on the ability to parent.

For example:

- Restricted amplitude and range of emotions might affect ability to empathise and sensitively respond to the baby's and older children's needs.

- Cognitive impairment might reduce ability to notice those needs.

- Withdrawal into one's own world increases the risk of emotional and physical neglect.

It is estimated that about half of women suffering from chronic schizophrenia will not be able to parent their children independently. The availability of consistent, long term support from other family members is a significant consideration when a legal decision is being made about a woman with chronic SMI's ability to parent.

It is important to differentiate psychosis as a part of SMI from that triggered by substance misuse or withdrawal from addictive substance, caused by physical problems (for example, infections) or occurring on the background of an acute psychosocial crisis in the context of personality difficulties. These problems might also overlap.

Assessing high risk presentations

As noted above under 'puerperal psychosis', psychotic symptoms can be associated with increased risk of harm to self and children. It is particularly important to remember this when the content of those symptoms refers to children. For example, a mother may have a delusion that her children are not hers or experience auditory hallucinations in the form of 'voice(s)' telling her to harm the children; she may lack insight as to the source of the voices, and could feel compelled to act on them. In this context, children may need to be separated temporarily from their mother and cared for by others in order to manage this risk, and the mother may require care from inpatient services or crisis and home treatment teams. Social services involvement should be considered, as per the local safeguarding children policy. Risk of self-harm, including risk of suicide, also needs to be considered.

In many cases these symptoms respond well to pharmacological treatment and an increased level of care for the time of their occurrence. Family members should be offered psycho-education and their worries listened to and discussed.

Identification and referral pathways for perinatal women with past or current severe mental illness

Midwives, health visitors and other health professionals who have contact with women in pregnancy and the postnatal period, play a vital role in the process of screening and possible identification of women with past and/or current SMI.

It is of course recommended that screening for mental health difficulties should be carried out in early pregnancy in order to allow as much time as possible for any further assessment and planning of care to meet the needs of the woman and her baby. The structured booking interview conducted by midwives at around 12 weeks gestation includes questions that ask women about current and/or past history of SMI (as recommended by CMACE, 2011 and NICE, 2014). These include:

- Asking about any past or present severe mental illness and past or present treatment by secondary or specialist mental health services, including inpatient care.

- Asking about a family history of perinatal SMI in a first degree relative, e.g. mother, sister or daughter. This can yield important information relating to increased risk of postpartum psychosis for women who have such a family history.

Additional questions are also useful in collating important information, such as:

- Current or past symptoms and the extent and nature of their impact on functioning.

- History relevant to mental health and any associated risks, for example:
  - risk to self – such as neglecting personal care, accidents, history of self-harm, and suicidal thoughts, intent or actions.
  - risk to others – such as harm or neglect.

Knowledge of past and/or current risk and context is vital as part of a comprehensive assessment of someone's mental health difficulties and essential for future risk prediction and further planning of care.

Case example: Emma

Emma first presented to mental health services when her first child was three months old. She was very depressed, and had developed negative thoughts that her daughter did not like her and that she was therefore a failure as a mother. She concluded that her daughter and everyone else would be better off without her, and she described to her health visitor planning a scenario where she would jump from a railway bridge to end her life.

Emma engaged with inpatient and outpatient mental health services for over a year, but was often quite guarded in how much she would reveal to health professionals regarding her suicidal thinking.

Asking questions inviting Emma to share her difficult feelings would allow an opportunity for her to share her negative thoughts, be offered timely support and services, and to hopefully reduce risk of harm.

Having conversations about difficult thoughts and feelings

Techniques for sensitively asking questions about risk and any other potentially difficult issues are invaluable for health professionals. A sympathetic, non-judgemental style is, of course, what we strive to achieve, and is also what we hope for from all health professionals we encounter ourselves. Normalising experiences often helps people to share information they might otherwise feel embarrassed or ashamed of. For example, this could be by asking:

'Many people, when they feel very down, lose hope and feel like doing anything to get away from their current difficulties. Have you ever felt this way?'

If someone responds affirmatively to this, additional questions can then be asked to explore this further.

The screening questions described above can serve as helpful tools for understanding a woman's mental health history and current/future needs. The information women give can be very useful when trying to gauge the possible nature and severity of any mental health difficulty, and whether referral to secondary or specialist mental health services should be considered.

Referral to a secondary or specialist mental health service should be made for women with past or current SMI:

- **When women are planning a pregnancy:** NICE (2014) recommend referral to specialist mental health services for pre-conception assessment, advice and support.

- **During pregnancy:** The referral should be made as early as possible in pregnancy or post-partum if not done before. NICE (2014) also recommend ensuring that a woman's GP is informed of the referral.

Women with a history of postpartum psychosis or bipolar disorder could have a 50% risk of developing a relapse of severe mood disorder or postpartum psychosis very soon after childbirth. This risk can be considered higher (up to 70%) in women who also have a family history of bipolar disorder or postpartum psychosis (NICE, 2014). We would recommend that the risk should not be considered to be significantly reduced even if women have remained well for a considerable length of time since their last episode of illness.

It is therefore recommended that secondary or perinatal mental health services undertake an assessment and monitoring during pregnancy and until at least three months after delivery, when the risk of postpartum psychosis is significantly lower.

Planning optimum care

It is also recommended that mental health services develop a perinatal care plan with the woman, which is distributed to relevant healthcare professionals with her consent, ideally by 28 weeks gestation. It is recommended that, if necessary, referrals to secondary care or specialist mental health services are made as early as possible in pregnancy. A referral should also be made in the postnatal period if not made earlier, for the reasons above.

Case example: Sasha

Sasha is pregnant with her first child, and was admitted to hospital with a psychotic episode two years ago. During her illness episode, Sasha responded to a visual hallucination of her mother (who was actually deceased in reality at the time) by running through a glass door to get to her, sustaining severe cuts to her arms and face.

Sasha's history may suggest that she is at a high risk of postpartum psychosis. Early referral to mental health services would be recommended. Services would aim to work with Sasha to create a plan of care, to ensure she receives the support necessary to reduce the risk of relapse (for many women this may include education regarding the importance of adequate sleep and how often sleep deprivation is a trigger for perinatal SMI) together with a plan that aims to ensure the safety of Sasha and her baby should she become unwell (for example, to ensure that sufficient support is available from family and professionals to recognise early relapse indicators, with a contingency plan to be brought into play should these emerge).

Making referrals

In general, referrals should be made in writing to the local general adult or perinatal community mental health team, subject to local variations in services and care pathways.

The urgency of referral and recommended response times differ depending on the woman's presentation. A non-urgent referral in writing can usually be made if the woman herself is mentally well.

If a woman's presentation suggests current SMI, an urgent referral should be made if in doubt. This can be done via telephone consultation to mental health services, supported by written information. NICE (2014) make recommendations regarding response times for assessment by mental health services. For a woman presenting with postpartum psychosis the recommended maximum time from referral to assessment is four hours.

Giving specific information in your referral

To communicate the need for services as well as possible within the referral, it is advisable to use specific examples regarding the woman's symptoms, the impact they are having on her functioning, and the risks to her, her children and others. The more specific the better; we have seen many referrals declined in the past, when services receive a referral with information which can be interpreted towards the milder end of the possible spectrum of severity if not explicit, for example, 'this woman is having difficulty coping' (see also Chapter 11: Challenges for midwives, on this point).

It is advisable to continuously update information held regarding local mental health services and referral routes in advance, as care pathways can vary according to area and change over time.

It is also important to follow the recommendations within NICE guidelines (2011; 2012) when making referrals, including some of the following principles.
It is important to discuss any potential referral to mental health services with the woman herself. Ensuring this is done well is invaluable, as it helps to foster

a collaborative alliance with the woman and creates an opportunity to discuss her thoughts, feelings and anxieties. Many women may be anxious about referral to mental health services owing to concerns about stigma. They may fear that information could be shared with children's social care, and that their parenting ability could be viewed as unsatisfactory because they have a mental health difficulty (NICE, 2014). Allowing a dialogue about these and any other anxieties is a crucial part of developing a shared understanding of a woman's concerns and offering appropriate reassurance.

It is also, of course, essential that all patients have sufficient information about potential decisions in order to make an informed choice. Every possible attempt should be made to obtain informed consent from a woman herself before making a referral to mental health services. This also includes obtaining consent to share information with other health professionals – for example, a GP, midwife or health visitor – to inform them that a referral has been made, for optimal communication and joined-up working.

Obtaining informed consent may not be possible if, for example, a woman declines the referral or accepts but lacks capacity regarding decision-making around this. In circumstances where women do not provide informed consent for referral, it is advisable to consult with colleagues as to how to proceed. It can be useful to discuss the case with seniors, safeguarding leads and mental health services. When seeking advice, this can be done without using patient-identifiable information if unsure that referral is justified. If a patient lacks capacity to consent, further assessment in concordance with the Mental Capacity Act (2005) may be required regarding acting in their best interests.

Further assessment within the framework of the Mental Health Act (2007) may be necessary if a patient's health or safety, or the safety of others, is at risk as a result of their mental disorder. For example, depression may be associated with suicidal ideas. Someone with severe mental illness, for example psychosis, may experience other symptoms which increase the risk to themselves or others, such as hearing voices (auditory hallucinations) commanding the person to do something harmful to themselves or others, or delusional beliefs (unshakeable false convictions) leading that person to believe they must act in a way that could in reality be of high risk to themselves or others.

A person with a mental disorder with a risk of marked neglect of self that significantly compromises their health or safety would also be considered for assessment under the Mental Health Act (2007).

Physical health

Always consider any possible physical health-related conditions precipitating or exacerbating factors regarding a woman's mental health presentation, for example, the possible role of thyroid dysfunction in mood disorder. The Centre for Maternal and Child Enquiries (CMACE) *Saving Mothers' Lives* report (2011) included a similar recommendation: that great caution needs to be exercised when making a diagnosis of a psychiatric disorder alone when the only symptoms are unexplained physical symptoms and distress or agitation. Many women have died in the perinatal period when serious medical conditions were missed because symptoms were presumed to be due to psychiatric issues in women already assigned a diagnosis of mental disorder. For example, a woman with pulmonary embolus died after presenting with anxiety, shortness of breath and palpitations, which were presumed to be due to anxiety alone as she was already diagnosed with an anxiety disorder.

After referral

Primary care professionals, including midwives and health visitors, can play a vital part in the continuity of care in their relationship with the woman, in support, and in liaison and communication with all other relevant health and social care professionals – with the woman's consent.

After referral, the woman should be offered an assessment with specialist mental health services. The assessment should lead to the development of a multidisciplinary multi-agency care plan stating the needs of the woman, any risks, and recommended treatments and services.

For women who are currently mentally unwell, consideration will need to be made regarding where the woman's care can be managed safely. Services should always aim to offer treatment in the least restrictive environment. This could be in the community, possibly with input from a home treatment or crisis team. If this cannot be managed safely, inpatient care may be necessary, which is often the case in severe perinatal mental illness.

It is recommended that for women needing mental health inpatient care (if they have an infant up to the age of one year), a mother and baby unit admission should be arranged (rather than a general adult inpatient admission without their infant) unless there is a specified reason for not doing so (NICE, 2014).

'MBUs are designed to address a number of challenges, including the need for specialist expertise in the treatment of severe perinatal illness, the need to support the development of the mother-infant relationship through a joint admission, and

the provision of an environment that is safe and appropriate to the care of a young infant (for example, the presence of specialist nursery nurses and the avoidance of the severe disturbance seen on many general inpatient wards) and to the physical needs of pregnant and postnatal women. The functions of inpatient services for women with mental health problems during pregnancy and the postnatal period include:

- *assessment of mental illness, including risk assessment and assessment of ability to care for the infant*

- *provision of expert care of women requiring admission*

- *in MBUs, the expert provision of safe care for the infants of women admitted*

- *support for the woman in caring for and developing a relationship with her baby, wherever appropriate fostering the involvement of the partner or other carers*

- *liaison and integrated working with other services, including maternity and obstetric services, GPs, and maternity-based and community mental health services.'*

(NICE, 2014)

Treatments

Treatments offered should address the biological-psychological-social predisposing, precipitating and maintaining factors for a woman's mental illness. Treatments offered could include the following.

Psychotropic medication

Psychotropic medication should be used in accordance with NICE (2014). It may include antipsychotic, mood stabilising and/or antidepressant medication. Short-term anxiolytic or hypnotic medication can also be offered.

In pregnant and breastfeeding women, decision-making around prescribing medication must always take into account the balance of risks and benefits involved, that is, risks to baby and benefits to the mother from treatment, versus longer term risks to the baby from ineffective treatment of the mother's mental disorder. Prescribers should always aim to select medication that poses the lowest known risks to the baby and use the minimum effective doses. Consideration must be made regarding potential and actual side effects – for example, sedation – which may interfere with functioning and parenting. Mothers should always be involved in treatment decisions and be given information in a variety of formats to enhance understanding.

Electroconvulsive therapy

Electroconvulsive therapy (ECT) is a biological intervention, which is used in cases of very severe mental illness where attempts at treatment using medication have been unsuccessful and/or rapid improvement is imperative.

Psychological interventions

These can be used in SMI and a lower threshold for offering these (compared to non-perinatal women) may be applied owing to the increased risks associated with medication in pregnancy or breastfeeding.

Various forms of psychological therapy can be offered, including cognitive behavioural therapy and psychodynamic psychotherapies, including parent-infant psychotherapy, where available.

Some centres – for example mother and baby units (MBUs) – may be able to conduct mother-infant relationship interventions, which are psychological interventions that aim to improve the relationship between the mother and infant. These are based on psychological theory about the nature of attachment between the mother and infant. They typically involve observations of mother-infant interactions, feedback (often video-based), modelling and cognitive restructuring. The primary aim is to enhance maternal sensitivity to child behavioural cues and awareness of the child's developing skills and needs (NICE, 2014).

Social interventions

Addressing social difficulties such as housing, finance, social isolation and lack of support can be of enormous benefit. Specific interventions can be directed at addressing any exacerbating or maintaining factors perpetuating the course of mental illness, for example, domestic violence.

Conclusion

Although severe mental illness presents an enormous challenge in the perinatal period and can be a very harrowing experience for women and their families, the goal of mental health services is to provide a positive experience of care for every woman to help her feel supported, safe and empowered on her journey to recovery with her infant and family. Health professionals from many disciplines can play a valuable role in helping women and their families to achieve this.

References

Centre for Maternal and Child Enquiries (CMACE) (2011) Saving mothers' lives: reviewing maternal deaths to make motherhood safer. *British Journal of Obstetrics and Gynaecology* **118** (Supplement 1) 1–203.

Kendell RE, Chalmers JC & Platz C (1987) Epidemiology of puerperal psychoses. *British Journal of Psychiatry* **150** 662–673.

National Institute for Health and Care Excellence (NICE) (2011) *Service User Experience in Adult Mental Health: Improving the experience of care for people using adult NHS mental health services* [online]. NICE clinical guideline 136. London: NICE. Available at: www.nice.org.uk/guidance/cg136 (accessed April 2016).

National Institute for Health and Care Excellence (NICE) (2012) *Patient Experience in Adult NHS Services: Improving the experience of care for people using adult NHS services.* NICE clinical guideline 138. London: NICE. Available at: www.nice.org.uk/guidance/cg138 (accessed April 2016).

National Institute for Health and Care Excellence (NICE) (2014) *Antenatal and Postnatal Mental Health: Clinical management and service guidance.* NICE clinical guideline 192. London: NICE. Available at: www.nice.org.uk/guidance/cg192 (accessed April 2016).

World Health Organization (1992) *The ICD-10 Classification of Mental and Behavioural Disorders.* Geneva: WHO.

Chapter 10: Other types of maternal mental health difficulties

Sue Gellhorn

The recognition of and attention to postnatal depression has been increasing in an encouraging fashion over the past few decades. In the context of these developments in academic and clinical arenas, women's voices in online forums and support organisations (for example, Netmums, Pandas Foundation) and the new campaign of the Maternal Mental Health Alliance (2014), much better recognition and appraisal of antenatal and postnatal anxiety has also arrived. The Bristol longitudinal studies (Evans *et al*, 2001) and the startling psychophysiological work of researchers such as Vivette Glover (Glover *et al*, 2010) have built up an evidence base for the understanding of the impact of maternal emotional states on the psychophysiology and development of unborn and newborn babies.

In addition to perinatal depression, antenatal and postnatal anxiety, and the more severe perinatal illnesses discussed in Chapter 9, there are a number of areas of difficulty that present rather differently and need to be better understood in order to be recognised in the maternity clinic or within postnatal and early mother baby care. The main areas of difficulty that will be covered in this chapter are:

- post-traumatic stress disorder
- obsessive-compulsive disorder
- social anxiety
- substance abuse and addictions
- personality disorder
- eating disorders.

Outlined in this chapter are some of the important features of these disorders, as well as some thoughts and findings about how professionals and community service providers can listen and talk to women with these difficulties, in order to help them in pregnancy and early motherhood.

Post-traumatic stress disorder (PTSD)

Post-traumatic stress disorder (PTSD) is an area of difficulty that is beginning to be much better recognised in maternity and mother-baby care settings. However, it is also often overlooked in favour of a vague assessment of 'depression' or 'anxiety', with the result that the most appropriate help or treatment is not made available. This section is intended to help in the identification of PTSD and the specific features of mental distress shown by women with this disorder.

There is a spectrum of post-traumatic stress, which includes:

■ a single episode adult trauma – such as having a car accident, or being mugged or assaulted – leading to a transitory traumatic reaction

■ developmental trauma leading to a variety of psychiatric manifestations in adulthood

■ complex trauma, including experiences of war crimes, torture and political persecution.

Definition

'Post-traumatic stress disorder occurs after a traumatic event that involved actual or threatened death or serious injury, or threat to the physical integrity of self or others. The affected person will have experienced intense fear, helplessness or horror when the event occurred.'
(Stubley, 2010)

Trigger events include physical, psychological or sexual abuse, terrorism and war, domestic violence, witnessing violence against others, accidents and natural disasters. Symptoms usually begin within three months of the incident but occasionally emerge years later, often following a further trigger event.

The symptoms of PTSD come under three main headings:

1. Re-experiencing phenomena.

2. Avoidance and numbing.

3. Increased arousal.

Examples of symptoms in these categories could include the following:

1. Recurrent and intrusive memories of the incident (sometimes called flashbacks) and dreams.

2. Avoiding discussion of or geographical proximity to the scene of an event.

3. Hyper-vigilance, difficulty sleeping and an exaggerated startle response.

The co-morbidity rates for PTSD are high. This means around 80% of women suffering PTSD will also be struggling with other sorts of difficulties, such as depression, an anxiety disorder, or substance misuse and dependence (Stubley, 2010).

Complex trauma

Many women of childbearing age have experienced complex trauma and many of these women will come for help in primary care, maternity services and children's centres. Many more will find it difficult to access services and to ask for help or give an account of their fears and difficulties. They may have tried every means possible to switch off their arousal, often resulting in them trying not to feel anything at all. These women need a particularly thoughtful and sensitive approach and may, more than ever, need to build up trusting relationships with professionals before the full extent of their needs becomes apparent.

Complex trauma includes experiences such as domestic violence, political torture, detention as a prisoner of war, living in transit and displacement as a refugee. Studies suggest that early experiences of childhood trauma may increase future vulnerability to trauma (see case example, Ardiana in Chapter 8). This of course links with our understanding of neurophysiological and attachment studies with infants. We know the impact of developmental trauma on resilience. We may often see this in the women on the delivery suite or at the baby clinic who find it most difficult to manage challenging experiences, such as an instrumental delivery or holding their baby while a nurse gives the baby an injection.

Vigilance to potential danger

The neurobiological model of trauma suggests that the impact event stimulates the thalamus, which is a subcortical structure involved in memory and experiences. The thalamus activates the amygdala, which results in autonomic nervous system responses, such as those seen in 'fight' or 'flight' responses. There will be a kind of vigilance to threat or danger and an autonomic over-drive, causing sweating, palpitations and stomach-churning symptoms.

This process happens without involvement of a second pathway to the thalamus, which can link to other areas of the brain called the cortex and hippocampus. This pathway allows for symbolisation and the laying down of a verbal memory. If events and experiences can be thought about involving verbal memory, the events can be given meaning and put into their historical and personal context. This means that such experiences then have a chance to be processed both emotionally and in words and integrated into a personal narrative.

In PTSD, flashbacks and reliving experiences are very frightening because they bring feelings of fear and threat that do not occur with a sense of time or context. These fears resemble the pre-verbal terrors of a baby who has not yet learned that bad experiences can be recovered from and made more manageable by comfort and support from another, the so-called 'nameless dread' (Bion, 1962).

Childbirth as a traumatic event

Childbirth is of course a very common event and as such is readily seen as 'normal' whatever form the experience takes. However, pregnancy, labour and delivery are challenging and stressful for many women. Case studies over the past 20 years have shown that women can suffer extreme psychological distress as a consequence of their experiences. For some women this is as the result of complications such as stillbirth or medical interventions that do not proceed as planned. Other women have what obstetrically might be recorded as a 'normal' birth but feel traumatised by aspects such as:

- loss of control
- loss of dignity
- the harsh or critical attitudes of the people around them.

It is now well recognised that it is not the objective severity of an event that determines the likelihood of PTSD but the woman's perception of events and her level of fear.

Currently there are no large scale research studies, but the evidence comes from case studies and in-depth interviews (Ford & Ayers, 2012). These show that women can suffer for years with PTSD symptoms after a difficult delivery experience. These symptoms, and particularly feelings of anger, can significantly affect a mother's relationship with her baby.

How maternity care can help

Women approaching pregnancy and birth with existing risk factors for PTSD (for example, a history of trauma, childhood sexual abuse or psychiatric problems) may need particular care to support them positively towards a life-affirming experience of birth. Evidence shows that interactions with others can have a strong impact on PTSD. Research shows that good support during labour and birth improves physical and psychological outcomes. Women who tell of feeling traumatised after birth often describe negative interactions with caregivers, such as feeling rushed, bullied, judged, ignored or put-off when asking for pain relief. See www.birthtraumaassociation.org for more information.

This is another example of the containing function of the caregiver towards the distress or uncertainty of another. Just as we hope the mother will come to be thoughtful towards her distressed infant and make efforts to understand, soothe and make manageable his or her pain, so we need to take steps to offer a labouring woman the sort of care where she will feel understood, listened to, and supported and reassured. As Gerhardt eloquently conveys in her book, secure relationships help us to regulate feelings, whether you are a young baby or an adult woman facing the challenge that is childbirth. She adds:

'Just holding the hand of someone you trust can reduce the activity of fear circuits in the brain.'
(Gerhardt, 2015, p160)

Screening and treatment

Currently there is no recognised screening tool for PTSD. Postnatally, without careful delineation of symptoms and history, many women with PTSD may be diagnosed with postnatal depression and given medication that is unlikely to prove an effective treatment. Treatment usually involves psychological therapy, either CBT or eye-movement desensitisation therapy (EMDR), both of which are recommended in NICE guidelines (2014)

A key part of recovery from these difficulties will involve talking about them. A sensitive conversation with a GP, midwife or health visitor about current fears and past experiences may be the first step in the recovery process.

Obsessive-compulsive disorder (OCD)

Obsessive-compulsive disorder during pregnancy and after having a baby has been given very little research attention despite being a significant mental health problem for many women. Some women develop OCD for the first time in the perinatal period, whereas others find a pre-existing condition becomes worse as they enter motherhood. There is also a strong possibility that OCD is under-diagnosed in the population generally, and the more intense health attention that women receive as part of maternity care, and, of course, women's concerns about the impact of OCD symptoms on their baby, means that symptoms may be more likely to be disclosed by women in the perinatal period (McGuiness *et al*, 2011). As a cause of perinatal mental ill-health, OCD is now thought to affect two to four per cent of all new mothers. See http://www.ocduk.org/prenatal-postnatal-ocd for more information about perinatal OCD.

In pregnancy and early parenthood women and their partners are naturally focused on the safety and well-being of their unborn and newborn child. They take on a responsibility like no other, and receive a proliferation of guidance and health recommendations about their baby's needs. Women are uniquely attuned to protecting their baby and acutely aware that their own actions have an immediate impact on their child. On top of this, the physical upheavals, general stress and role adjustments can make it challenging for many new parents to feel confident and relaxed.

Definition

'Obsessive-compulsive disorder is an anxiety disorder characterised by recurrent, unwelcome thoughts, ideas, doubts or images (obsessions) that give rise to distress and urges to respond to this obsessional anxiety with excessive behavioural or mental acts (compulsions).'
(Abramowitz *et al*, 2003, p462)

Some experts are of the view that perinatal OCD presents a distinct clinical picture and it does seem that the content or obsessions at this time focus on the parent's fear of purposely harming their newborn baby or somehow being responsible for accidental harm.

Many new parents experience fleeting thoughts of this nature, so in one sense they are normal and very common. However, some people are so disturbed by them that they will go to considerable lengths to manage their anxiety and take preventative steps so that 'nothing bad can happen'. Thus it is the extent of the worries and the mother's response to them that define the mental health problem.

Recognising perinatal OCD

Examples of obsessional thoughts focusing on infant harm include:

- fear of harming the baby from impact with hard surfaces or sharp objects

- recurrent thoughts of the baby dying in his or her sleep, or contracting disease

- worries about inadvertently or deliberately sexually abusing the baby

- thoughts of throwing the baby downstairs or out of a window

- worries that the baby might be left behind somewhere.

'I keep thinking I'm going to hurt him. Something terrible is going to happen. I see myself picking up a knife or holding his head under water.'
(A new mother speaking about obsessional thoughts, Kleiman, 2009, p158)

Examples of compulsions in response to obsessional thoughts and images include:

- compulsive rituals (behaviour), such as repeated washing, sterilising or checking

- compulsive covert rituals, such as counting, rehearsing or 'neutralising' thoughts

- avoidance of obsessional 'cues', such as knives or bathing the baby, or avoidance of general contact with the baby.

Case example: Hannah

Hannah was a down-to-earth charity administrator who had her first child in her mid-30s. Keen to have more children, she became pregnant with her second child more quickly than expected. On her second maternity leave she found the competing demands of her active toddler son and her newborn daughter challenging. Always a worrier who set herself high standards, she began to have very disturbing thoughts about harming her newborn. She saw vivid images of herself holding a knife over her baby's cot. For a while she managed to cope by spending almost all her daytime hours in the company of other mothers. This was both reassuring and exhausting. She also took the step of putting her sharp knives well out of reach. She had been pleased to give up smoking in her first pregnancy but found she could only cope in the hour or so she was alone with the children before her husband got home by taking herself to the bottom of the garden with a cigarette.

Eventually, she felt so bad about herself and the distancing effect her symptoms were having on her relationship with her new baby that she took her worries to her GP. When the GP asked if she was having thoughts that were worrying her it was both terrifying and a huge relief to reveal the thoughts that had become such a torment and finally get some help.

Because of the graphic content of many obsessional thoughts, they cause considerable anxiety, both for the women themselves and healthcare providers that they come into contact with. Women may try many strategies to suppress or distract themselves from their distressing thoughts; these are often unsuccessful, however, and seeking reassurance often also fails to bring relief. Because women with OCD have the insight that these thoughts are their own, they find them even more disturbing and the woman will often feel that such thoughts indicate she is either going mad or are a bad mother or both.

Supporting women seeking help with such difficulties is important, as it is now understood that many people hide their OCD symptoms for a considerable period of time. It is also important to note that in one study, 70% of women with OCD reported a dysfunctional relationship with their infant because of 1) avoidance of the infant, 2) fear about separation from their infant or 3) feeling fearful of allowing others to care for their infant (McGuiness *et al*, 2011).

Helpful things to say to women with perinatal OCD

Women are aware that their thoughts are irrational and do not reflect the way they feel about their baby. In psychiatry this is referred to as ego-dystonic, that is to say that such thoughts are not characteristic of who the woman is and are inconsistent with her desires or beliefs. For women with OCD, although such thoughts are deeply disturbing, they are rarely acted upon.

It may be helpful to explain the following to women with perinatal OCD:

- Having scary thoughts is very common.

- Telling a professional or someone else about the thoughts will not turn them into reality or make them happen.

- These thoughts are symptoms of an anxiety disorder called OCD.

- Having such troubling thoughts can feel like you are losing your mind. A common response is to try to stop thinking the distressing thoughts. Unfortunately, strong efforts to resist them can have the effect of reinforcing them.

The professional listening and containment offered at the point of disclosure of OCD can be extremely therapeutic and helpful. It is very helpful to reassure the woman that having bad thoughts does not mean she is a bad mother, and to let her know that talking about it and having treatment will help. Although the content of perinatal obsessions can be quite startling, it is important to avoid responding to a woman with obvious alarm; however, nor should she be reassured that such thoughts are completely normal, as the level of distress and shame she is experiencing will show her that they are not (Kendall-Tackett, 2010).

Understanding maternal ambivalence

Kleiman (2009) notes that in society we rarely consider that mothers might have thoughts of hurting their babies. It feels completely at odds with the images portrayed of motherhood in the media, in health promotion and in literature. Because of our somewhat idealised picture of how a mother should be, it seems impossible to believe that a mother might think or feel like this. Psychotherapists, in particular Parker (2005), have explored the nature of the conflicts behind maternal ambivalence. Parker also noted that while a great deal of psychoanalytic theory examines infants and their development, very little considers motherhood in depth and the impact of infants on mothers' perceptions of themselves.

Thinking about maternal ambivalence helps us understand the roots of perinatal OCD. Many everyday upsets can make a woman feel she is a bad mother, but one of the most powerful is feeling angry and resentful towards her baby. Culturally, women expect to feel angry with their adolescent children who are engaged in the process of separating and becoming independent. But it is much more difficult for mothers to feel comfortable with their angry feelings towards their dependent infant child. In psychoanalytic terms, OCD represents a situation where angry and hostile feelings are too shocking to the mother to be accepted as part of the myriad of emotional responses to her baby, and are actively pushed away.

We can see that well supported and less neurotic mothers, who are not so hard on themselves, are able to appreciate some distance and healthy separation from their babies from time to time. Such mothers, often those who are very well supported by family or close friends, are able to enjoy a break from their baby for a night out and restorative adult company.

Social anxiety disorder

Social anxiety disorder is one of a group of anxiety disorders that cause significant distress and interfere with everyday functioning. When anxiety is present at this level and is provoked by particular objects or situations, it is often referred to as 'phobic anxiety'. This contrasts with difficulties characterised as generalised anxiety disorder (sometimes referred to as GAD) where there is pervasive anxiety present across a range of life situations and settings. Social anxiety disorder was previously known in the field of mental health as 'social phobia'.

Definition

Social anxiety disorder is persistent fear of or anxiety about one or more social or performance situations. The level of anxiety is out of proportion to the actual threat of the situation.

People with social anxiety disorder often experience physical symptoms such as blushing, sweating, trembling and nausea. The anticipatory anxiety about these symptoms also creates difficulties. People with social anxiety often fear they will do or say something that will be humiliating or embarrassing, for example being lost for words or appearing stupid.

Common situations that provoke anxiety include: meeting new people, speaking in meetings or groups, eating out and formal social occasions, such as weddings and funerals. For further information about social anxiety/social phobia see http://www.mothersmatter.co.nz/Related-Conditions/Anxiety/Social-Phobia.asp and http://www.mind.org.uk.

While anxiety in some of these situations is common, the level of anxiety experienced by those with the disorder interferes significantly with everyday functioning, impacting on study and work performance, social relationships and quality of life. Avoidance of feared social situations is very common and in addition people often use alcohol and drugs to try to manage their anxiety.

Perinatal social anxiety

Social anxiety disorder tends to be under-recognised by GPs. Where it exists alongside depression, it is very common for the depression to be diagnosed and treated without the social anxiety disorder being picked up (see case example Christina on p141). In pregnancy, women are examined and assessed on a regular basis and asked questions about their health and their plans for parenthood. This attention can feel unwelcome and intensely uncomfortable for women with social anxiety. Many women feel that their parenting skills may be judged by others when they are out with their baby. For women with social anxiety, this can be experienced as acutely stressful. Breastfeeding is also often jeopardised by social anxiety disorder. Ordinary concerns about feeling conspicuous feeding a baby in public become, for a mother with social anxiety disorder, repeated episodes of acute stress and anxiety. This may mean breastfeeding cannot then be established or maintained.

Women with symptoms of social anxiety may have had these difficulties for a long time. For some women, focusing on the needs of their developing baby helps them tackle their anxieties. However, social anxiety can add a pressure to pregnancy and child-rearing that makes the challenges of motherhood feel overwhelming. For some new mothers, the pressures of their social anxiety mean that they severely limit the time they spend outside the home and become very socially isolated or dependent on family members. They may miss out on key services and opportunities for themselves and their baby. Improving symptoms and reducing avoidance behaviour is unlikely to be possible without lots of support and possibly professional intervention and treatment.

Case example: Christina

Christina's second daughter was born as a result of an unplanned pregnancy with her new partner. She had been working in a solicitor's office and after the birth she missed the structure and adult company of office life. When the baby was five months old, her partner got some well-paid contract work away from home and was unable to offer practical support with the baby during the week. Christina was worried about her teenage daughter, her energy levels became very low and she found it increasingly difficult to go out, feeling that other mothers in her local area were judging her. Her GP, who had known her for a number of years, asked her questions to assess her mood and felt she was depressed and becoming very isolated. She prescribed antidepressants and suggested referral to a local Family Action project which would help her get out of the house. At first Christina declined a visit from Family Action, but when the antidepressants helped improve her motivation she agreed to accept their input.

Substance abuse and addictions

Most women have an awareness that drugs taken in pregnancy particularly, but also when breastfeeding, present a potential risk of ill-health and harm to their baby. Sadly, despite these widespread protective intentions, many women who become pregnant are taking illicit substances and continue to do so despite their pregnancy. Substance misuse in pregnancy often coexists with a range of other problems, such as low income, poor quality housing and limited support networks. As a result, a number of care and support services are likely to be needed to promote good outcomes for the woman and her baby. Women who misuse substances are also more likely to have a history of abuse or neglect, to have negative experiences of parenting in their own childhoods and to have more negative representations of their unborn baby (Underdown & Barlow, 2012). For this group of women, pregnancies are less likely to be planned and co-morbidity of depression, anxiety and eating disorders is more common (Suchman *et al*, 2005).

The size of the population of drug-abusing mothers and mothers to be is difficult to measure. Two factors contribute to this uncertainty around prevalence of difficulties. The first is the fact that women will under-report their difficulty because of feelings of shame and fear of stigmatisation. Second, there is a frequent failure on the part of health professionals to enquire about drug use or recognise drug dependency.

Knowing that substances are harmful to the unborn child is often a powerful motivator for a woman to address her drug problem, and midwives and other health professionals have a crucial role in supporting women to access help.

Pregnancy disclosure

Studies have found that the situation of concealed pregnancy is more common in women who abuse drugs. Late presentation to healthcare services is very common in this group of mothers. There is often a misconception among class A drug-users that conception and pregnancy are unlikely if you are using heroin. Once women are aware of their pregnancy, medical services are often avoided through a combination of shame and fear.

Working with pregnant women who abuse substances

The Royal College of Midwives recommends the following approaches when working with pregnant women who misuse substances:

- Be available to listen, talk, understand and support.

- Ask women about substance/alcohol use sensitively, when the partner is not present, and provide multiple opportunities for disclosure.

- Provide flexible midwifery appointments and venues, and assurance that information will be confidential and not included in hand-held notes.

- Offer support from a dedicated substance/alcohol misuse support worker.

- Contribute to the development of clear local protocols/referral pathways in consultation with social care and voluntary sector providers.

- Support should also involve referral to social services for an appropriate pre-birth assessment and intervention.

(Underdown & Barlow, 2012)

Impact on early parenting and attachment

Parental drug misuse during the postnatal period will have a significant impact on the early experiences of the baby. The reality is that around 25% of children subject to a child protection plan will have a parent who is misusing substances (ACMD, 2004). Studies of parent-infant interaction where parents have these difficulties have observed emotional unavailability, incongruent mirroring and dysregulation in the mother-baby pair. These experiences affect the infant's developing nervous system and his or her capacity for emotional regulation later in childhood.

Other research has shown that substance abusing parents show a 'lack of understanding about basic child development issues, ambivalent feelings about having and keeping their children and less capacity to reflect on their baby's emotional and cognitive experience' (Suchman *et al*, 2005).

Alcohol abuse

Recommendations about alcohol consumption in pregnancy are becoming more strict than earlier guidance about limiting intake to one or two drinks. Guidance in the US, Australia and many other countries is to abstain altogether during pregnancy, as no safe level of drinking for the foetus has been established. Of course, for women who are regular heavy or binge drinkers this can be difficult to achieve. Regular alcohol use or binge drinking after the implantation stage has been shown to be harmful and is associated with foetal alcohol syndrome.

Pregnancy and having a baby are stressful times for women and their partners. Some women will have been in the habit of using alcohol as a coping mechanism before pregnancy and may continue to do so after pregnancy. However, alcohol is a depressant drug and can have an after-effect of increasing anxiety levels. Some of the negative outcomes of excessive alcohol use for new parents are:

- increased conflict with partners and family
- interference with early bonding with their baby
- impaired judgement, for example, about what is safe for babies
- sleepiness
- disinhibition and irritability.

Helping women think and talk about their alcohol use

Maternity and community professionals who are aware of alcohol problems in pregnant women and new mothers can take the following steps to promote safety and health for the woman and her baby:

- Help her think about the question, 'Do I have a problem with alcohol?'

- Help her think about whether the following apply to her drinking behaviour:

  - Is she binge drinking?

  - Is she dependent on alcohol (i.e. she cannot easily control the amount)?

  - Is she neglecting her responsibilities – for example, missing work/letting people down – because of alcohol?

  - How much salience does alcohol have in her life? Is getting alcohol and drinking often the main focus for her?

Women who clearly have a problem with alcohol or who show signs of developing one should be encouraged to make contact with alcohol services, especially services focused on the care of women. There are many safeguarding issues for women with alcohol problems. In particular, it is very difficult for such women to:

- put the needs of her unborn baby or new baby first

- accept that it is not safe to look after children in an intoxicated state

- make sure that their baby is put to bed safely if they have been drinking and, in particular, not to share a bed with them if they have been drinking.

Personality disorder

Identifying and sensitively helping women with a personality disorder can be a difficult business. For a considerable period of time, people with personality disorders were considered 'untreatable' by the psychiatric profession because their difficulties were seen as part of their personality as opposed to a mental disorder. This is no longer the case, and there has been helpful progress in the sort of therapy, support and clinical management that is now offered by mental health services (see, for example, www.emergenceplus.org.uk).

Definitions

The defining feature of a person who might come to be diagnosed with a personality disorder is that they have repeated and maladaptive patterns of perceiving and responding to other people in stressful situations. These patterns of behaviour represent rather rigid attempts at self-preservation, which tend not to shift in the face of advice and feedback from others. Typically, people with a personality disorder will make inaccurate attributions of feelings, thoughts and attitudes to others, especially when they are stressed or under pressure in some way. When these features of behaviour are assessed as longstanding, disabling and distressing, psychiatrists may make a diagnosis of personality disorder. There are a number of complex distinctions and categories, including paranoid personality disorder, antisocial personality disorder and borderline personality disorder (Hanley, 2009).

Borderline personality disorder in maternity settings

Perhaps the most common personality disorder that may be seen in maternity settings is that of borderline personality disorder. This may be because there is something of a bias in diagnosing this category in women or because there is an identified link with childhood abuse, especially sexual abuse, and women are more often victims of this sort of abuse. As adults, these women have a pattern of instability in their personal relationships coupled with reports of self-loathing and low self-esteem. They often seem to be involved in very intense interpersonal relationships where they either idealise or devalue the other. They may make frantic efforts to avoid being abandoned by people they are involved with. Sudden and dramatic shifts in their perception of others are very common. Self-harm is also very common and is used as a crude way of managing intense emotional reactions.

Women with borderline personality disorder find it very difficult to maintain relationships and in maternity settings may present with multiple pregnancies to different partners and sometimes multiple terminations of pregnancy too. Such women may present as very needy, demanding and distressed in maternity clinic settings. They can find it very difficult to manage their anxiety in their newly pregnant state and in an unfamiliar medical setting. They may become irritable and rude as their anxiety heightens.

It is worth remembering that these sorts of feelings and reactions are common to us all and that there is a continuum of disturbed responses to stress under extreme pressure. We can all be abrupt and irritable when we are highly anxious or fearful. It is important to keep these sensibilities to the fore when dealing with women who may have been given such a diagnosis.

Thinking about disordered personality presentations in child-bearing women links directly to the ideas and concepts in earlier chapters about attachment and emotional regulation in babies (see Chapter 4). Borderline personality disorder is seen in current thinking as a disorder of emotional regulation. So we can see that these mothers, who may be difficult to support and treat, are likely to have suffered deprivation as a baby and young child. They are likely to have lacked the support of a parent to help them regulate their emotions and learn about recovery from upset in a straightforward way. This results in an adult who is often in a highly stressed and emotional state. So we can see that having a personality disorder will add to the usual emotional tasks and social adjustment that parenthood brings.

Working with women with personality disorder

Just as there are frequent misunderstandings with partners, friends and family members for these women, there are often upsets and perceived slights and misunderstandings in their dealings with healthcare professionals. A difficulty making use of advice and professional help is a characteristic of women with borderline personality disorder. Services are now much better informed about helpful approaches for personality disorder but the 'label' can too readily be seen as indicating that a woman will be an unfit parent when this will need to be fully assessed postnatally when support that may be needed can be put in place. NICE (2014) recommends using the clinical case management approach for caring for women with a known personality disorder. However, there is currently little evidence base for the kinds of support and treatment that may best help new mothers with personality disorder difficulties and their partners to parent positively.

Eating disorders

There is a significant degree of concealment and shame surrounding eating disorders in the perinatal period. Like women with substance abuse problems, women may not readily reveal their difficulties in pregnancy, particularly if they see themselves as having been well for some time. An eating disorder has other parallels with substance abuse, as difficult feelings come to be managed habitually through a secret addiction that brings short-term release from distress.

There is a general expectation that women only become pregnant when recovered from an eating disorder. However, a sizeable number of women with eating disorders do become pregnant, and many of these may be women who have undergone fertility treatment who may not have revealed their eating disorder. Many young women with active bulimia symptoms assume their fertility is low and may have unplanned pregnancies as a result (Fawkner, 2012).

Definitions

Anorexia nervosa

The criteria for diagnosis are:

- The woman shows refusal to maintain appropriate body weight for her age and height.
- Despite low body weight, she demonstrates extreme anxiety about weight gain.
- She shows evidence of a distorted body image.
- Post-puberty, women and girls with the disorder may have amenorrhea (absence of menstruation).

Bulimia nervosa

The criteria for diagnosis are:

- Sufferers engage in periodic and sometimes ritualised binge eating.
- Calorie intake and weight are managed through intermittent meal restriction, self-induced vomiting or purging with laxatives.
- Like women with anorexia, they show distorted self-perceptions of their size and a predominant concern over weight and body shape.

Eating disorders and pregnancy

Pregnancies to women with eating disorders show a number of negative health outcomes, including:

- a higher rate of miscarriage
- a higher rate of prematurity
- more deliveries involving caesarean section or induction.

In extreme cases there may be multiple miscarriages or abortions induced by severe restriction of food and excessive exercise.

An eating disorder can delay detection of pregnancy and have a negative impact on health outcomes through delayed antenatal care. Women with eating disorders will display a range of psychological difficulties, from mild to quite a severe degree of disturbance. It is important to recognise that an eating disorder is not a lifestyle choice but is indicative of significant psychological disorder. There is a strong association between a history of sexual abuse and eating disorders. Both areas of difficulty would present challenges for a woman approaching motherhood. The Royal College of Psychiatrists (2012), for all of these reasons, recommends that where an eating disorder is detected in pregnancy, the woman is referred to mental health services for assessment.

There is some evidence that, postnatally, a mother with an eating disorder will be compromised in her mother-baby relationship, her nutritional care of her baby and her capacity to prioritise her baby's needs above her own. NICE (2014) make the following recommendations for psychological intervention in pregnancy or the postnatal period:

- Offer psychological treatment for the eating disorder.

- Monitor the woman's condition carefully throughout pregnancy and postnatally.

- Assess the need for foetal growth scans.

- Discuss the importance of healthy eating during pregnancy and postnatally.

- Advise the woman about feeding her baby (in accordance with guidance on maternal and child nutrition).

References

Abramowitz JS, Schwartz SA, Moore KM & Luenzmann KR (2003) Obsessive-compulsive symptoms in pregnancy and the puerperium: a review of the literature. *Journal of Anxiety Disorders* 17: 461–478.

Advisory Council on the Misuse of Drugs (ACMD) (2004) *Advisory Council on the Misuse of Drugs: Annual report, accounting year 2003–4*. London: Home Office.

Bion WR (1962) A theory of thinking. *International Journal of Psychoanalysis* **43** 306–310.

Evans J, Heron J, Francomb H, Oke S & Golding J (2001) Cohort study of depressed mood during pregnancy and after childbirth. *British Medical Journal* **323** (7307) 257–2601.

Fawkner H (2012) Eating disorders. In: C Martin (Ed) *Perinatal Mental Health: A clinical guide*. Keswick: M&K Publishing.

Ford E & Ayers S (2012) Post-traumatic stress disorder following childbirth. In: C Martin (Ed) *Perinatal Mental Health: A clinical guide*. Keswick: M&K Publishing.

Gerhardt S (2015) *Why Love Matters: How affection shapes a baby's brain* (2nd edition). Hove: Routledge.

Glover V, O'Connor TG & O'Donnell K (2010) Prenatal stress and the programming of the HPA axis. *Neuroscience and Behavioural Reviews* **35** (1) 17–22.

Hanley J (2009) *Perinatal Mental Health: A guide for health professionals and users*. Chichester:

Wiley-Blackwell.

Kendall-Tackett KA (2010) *Depression in New Mothers. Causes, consequences and treatment alternatives*. London: Routledge.

Kleiman K (2009) *Therapy and the Postpartum Woman: Notes on healing postpartum depression for clinicians and women who seek their help*. New York: Routledge.

Maternal Mental Health Alliance (2014) *Maternal Mental Health. Everyone's business* [online]. Available at: http://maternalmentalhealthalliance.org.uk/ (accessed April 2016).

McGuiness M, Blisset J & Jones C (2011) OCD in the perinatal period: Is postpartum OCD (ppOCD) a distinct subtype? A review of the literature. *Behavioural and Cognitive Psychotherapy* **39** (3) 285–310.

NICE (2014) *Antenatal and Postnatal Mental Health: Clinical management and service guidance* [online]. Available at: https://www.nice.org.uk/guidance/cg192 (accessed April 2016).

Parker R (2005) *Torn in Two: The experience of maternal ambivalence*. London: Virago.

Royal College of Psychiatrists (2012) *Perinatal Mental Health Difficulties* [self-help leaflet]. London: RCP.

Stubley J (2010) Post-traumatic stress disorder. In: D Kohen (Ed) *Oxford Textbook of Women and Mental Health*. Oxford: Oxford University Press.

Suchman NE, McMahon TJ, Slade A & Luthar SS (2005) How early bonding, depression, illicit drug use and perceived support work together to influence drug-dependent mothers' caregiving. *American Journal of Orthopsychiatry* **75** (3) 431–445.

Underdown A & Barlow J (2012) *Maternal Emotional Wellbeing and Infant Development: A good practice guide for midwives* [online]. London: Royal College of Midwives. Available at: www.rcm.org.uk/sites/default/files/Emotional%20Wellbeing_Guide_WEB.pdf (accessed January 2016).

Web resources

Birth Trauma Association: www.birthtraumaassociation.org.uk

Emergence: www.emergenceplus.org.uk

OCD-UK: www.OCDUK.org

Royal College of Psychiatrists (2012) *Mental Health in Pregnancy* [information leaflet]. Available at: www.rcpsych.ac.uk/healthadvice/problemsdisorders/mentalhealthinpregnancy.aspx (accessed January 2016).

Chapter 11: Challenges for midwives

Heather Jenkins

Introduction

Midwives face a variety of challenges on a daily basis. Meeting the needs of women and their families within the context of a rising birth rate, complex physical, psychological and social needs, and an NHS that struggles to provide adequate resources can be hugely demanding. Midwives are frequently under pressure to provide safe, compassionate and holistic care of the highest quality in circumstances that are often less than ideal.

Supporting women through their physical and psychological transition to motherhood is at the very heart of the midwife's role (MMHA *et al*, 2013). Indeed, midwives are uniquely placed to offer early interventions that will optimise the health outcomes for women and their families. Perinatal mental health is now a significant public health issue. It is thought that mental illness costs the UK £8.1 billion per year (Bauer *et al*, 2014). The most recent report into maternal deaths in the UK demonstrates that perinatal mental illness is one of the leading causes of death (Knight *et al*, 2015). One in seven late deaths (maternal deaths between six weeks and one year post birth) were due to suicide, which accounts for 23% of the total number of maternal deaths. The number of maternal deaths due to mental illness has remained consistently high while 'direct' causes of death such as haemorrhage and eclampsia have reduced in recent times. It is significant that resources are directed towards managing the physical risks to women during childbirth, yet the risks posed by mental illness are yet to be fully addressed.

Perinatal mental illness has a potentially devastating impact on women and their families. Midwives are very aware of this and there is palpable anxiety around this issue within the profession. This anxiety is exacerbated by media coverage of women whose mental health needs have not been met, resulting in tragedy. The very recent deaths of a mother and her baby in Bristol serve as an example of this (Morris, 2015).

Midwives are in a unique position to identify, assess and refer women when they begin to experience mental illness. Midwives are also able to promote mental health through supporting women to bond with their baby during pregnancy and immediately following birth, and continuing this support into the postnatal period (Underdown & Barlow, 2012). The importance of this cannot be overstated and is key to optimising both the woman's emotional well-being and that of her baby, who can then develop a secure attachment to his mother and thus ensure optimum development.

However, the issue of addressing a woman's mental health poses unique challenges to the midwife. This chapter will seek to discuss these and suggest ways that midwives can meet these challenges.

Challenge 1: Training

The NICE clinical guideline for antenatal and postnatal mental health states that:

'All healthcare professionals providing assessment and interventions for mental health problems in pregnancy and the postnatal period should understand the variations in their presentation and course at these times, how these variations affect treatment, and the context in which they are assessed and treated (for example, maternity services, health visiting and mental health services).'
(NICE, 2014)

This assumes a level of competence from the midwife, who is uniquely placed to identify and assess a woman's mental health through pregnancy and the postnatal period. This presents a challenge as recent evidence suggests that midwifery training in perinatal mental health is inadequate.

Of the 42,976 midwives currently registered with the Nursing & Midwifery Council (NMC, 2016), only five hold a dual registration of Registered Midwife (RM) and Registered Nurse in Mental Health (RNMH). This equates to 0.01% of midwives who are trained as midwives and mental health nurses. Of course, there will be midwives who hold qualifications in counselling or who may have a background in psychology, but this is not recognised by the profession's governing body. It is an interesting point that the dual RM/RNMH qualification is not a common career path for midwives.

Therefore, the majority of midwives are reliant on their intrinsic interest in a woman's psychological readiness and adjustment to motherhood and the pre- and post-registration training that they receive.

Pre-registration training

Current pre-registration midwifery training programmes are developed in accordance with the guidance set out in the 2009 Standards for Pre-Registration Midwifery Education (Nursing and Midwifery Council, 2009). In general, the courses do incorporate a psychological component for each of the topics covered and are developed with sensitivity to the issues surrounding mental health. Some universities include a module on perinatal mental health. However, more could be done to optimise this training. At this time, there is no mandatory requirement for perinatal mental health to be included in pre-registration midwifery training and there is no national guidance regarding course content that would ensure a uniformity of the quantity and quality of training for student midwives (Hogg, 2013; MMHA, 2014; RCM, 2014).

A recent survey of student midwives reported that:

- 24.1% did not feel well enough trained in issues around mental health

- 26.7% did not feel confident to recognise the signs of mental illness.

(RCM, 2014)

This should be compared with a study in 2006, where 29% of midwives said that they had received no mental health training in their pre-registration programme. Of the 71% that had received training, 17.6% stated that it was insufficient (Ross-Davie *et al*, 2006). It would seem that little has changed in the provision of adequate training in perinatal mental health for pre-registration student midwives despite increased awareness of the impact these health issues can have on women and their families.

The lack of adequate pre-registration training creates a midwifery workforce which is under-confident in identifying, assessing and referring women who are experiencing mental health difficulties. This has potentially huge implications for the women and their families. It is significant that the lack of training opportunities for student midwives is mirrored by a lack of post-registration training for qualified midwives.

Post-registration training

Midwives must receive regular updates of their clinical skills and knowledge so that they can offer safe and effective care to women. However, training in perinatal mental health is often omitted or minimalised when there are competing topics that need to be incorporated into a training programme. The NSPCC gathered information from NHS trusts in England to assess the quality and quantity of mental health training for qualified midwives (Hogg, 2013). The study showed that:

- 10% of trusts reported that no midwife had received any training on perinatal mental health in the past year

- 68% of trusts stated that their midwifery staff are required to do some training in perinatal mental health

- 50% of these trusts stated that it is mandatory for midwives to undertake annual training in perinatal mental health.

It seems clear that NHS trusts need to work harder to incorporate perinatal mental health within their annual mandatory midwifery training.

It is also clear that there needs to be national guidance around how the training is delivered and by whom, such as the Curricular Framework used in Scotland (NHS Education for Scotland, 2006). In this Scottish guidance, a comprehensive curriculum is given and key competencies for different staff groups are specified. In their research the NSPCC noted that training in perinatal mental health for midwives often lasted less than an hour, consisted of a set of PowerPoint slides and was often included in sessions that covered safeguarding and related issues, such as domestic abuse and substance misuse. Given that perinatal mental health is such a significant public health issue, it would seem that this is not sufficient and it needs dedicated training time in its own right.

The NSPCC, RCM and Maternal Mental Health Alliance make the following recommendations (Hogg, 2013; MMHA, 2014; RCM, 2014):

- Post-registration training for midwives should be offered, ideally by a specialist perinatal mental health midwife.

- If this is not possible, training should be delivered by someone who is trained and experienced in perinatal mental health.

Training for midwives should include:

- how to identify the risk factors for perinatal mental illness, including the Whooley questions and the Generalized Anxiety Disorder Scale (GAD-2) (NICE, 2014)

- the identification and management of the full range of mental health issues that women may experience

- methods of making a referral within the local care pathway for perinatal mental health

- medication, including the implications for breastfeeding and the impact on the foetus/neonate

- how to identify safeguarding concerns and refer appropriately

- an opportunity for midwives to discuss any cases of concern or to role play in order to build confidence and skills in communication.

The quality and the quantity of the training is very important if midwives are to be supported in developing their skills and knowledge in this area. Communication skills are a key area in all midwifery practice, but especially crucial in maternal mental health, where having conversations with women about difficult feelings is key.

The lack of post-registration university modules in perinatal mental health is also significant. If most NHS trusts are offering inadequate training and there are limited options in terms of courses run by universities, how are midwives able to develop their knowledge and awareness? There are training options available online (NSPCC, 2012; RCM, n.d.) and Local Safeguarding Children Boards (LSCBs) will provide training on the impact of parental mental illness on the child. There are also a considerable number of study days and forums run by external organisations that focus on perinatal mental health. However, there are many factors that may present obstacles for the midwife to engage with these. For example, each of these options would probably have to be undertaken in a midwife's spare time, as a busy NHS trust may prove reluctant to release staff for a study day when there is pressure to achieve safe staffing levels within the maternity unit. It is also unlikely in the current climate that an NHS trust would fund such study sessions unless the midwife were to go to considerable lengths to justify the value of the training to management. Furthermore, there is already a huge demand on midwives for their study time (Rowan *et al*, 2010). The move towards mandatory training via e-learning often results in midwives making personal efforts to complete online training sessions, frequently in their own time. It is therefore hugely challenging for the midwife to develop their knowledge and skills in the provision of perinatal mental healthcare. However, there is hope for the future. As part of the government's current commitment to addressing the impact of perinatal mental health, they have pledged that all midwives will receive training in mental health (MMHA *et al*, 2013; DH, 2013; BPS, 2014; Press Association, 2014). At the time of writing, this promise also forms part of the opposition party's plan. This feels reassuring and is certainly reflective of the recommendations made by several key organisations (MMHA *et al*, 2013; Hogg, 2013; MMHA, 2014; RCM, 2014). Furthermore, the Royal College of Midwives has published a clear standard and competencies framework for midwives who specialise in perinatal mental health (RCM, 2015). Increased access to quality training in perinatal mental health for midwives will directly increase the opportunities for early identification, assessment and appropriate referral by confident and competent midwives. This will directly improve the outcomes for women and their families.

Organisational challenges

Research suggests that only 30% of women who experience mental health issues share their feelings with a healthcare professional (Boots Family Trust *et al*, 2013). It is really useful for midwives to reflect on this statistic and consider what barriers there are to women disclosing their feelings in an honest and open way. Many of these barriers exist because of organisational challenges that need to be addressed in order to open up the relationship between the midwife and the woman and make disclosure of mental health issues feel safe.

Challenge 2: Continuity of care

Continuity of care has been a central concept within the provision of midwifery care for many years and is widely recognised as one of the key factors in optimising the experience and outcomes of women throughout pregnancy, childbirth and the postnatal period (Sandall, 2014; DH, 1993). It also enhances the feeling of job satisfaction for midwives. The NICE guidelines for antenatal care, pregnancy and complex social factors and antenatal and postnatal mental health (CG 62, CG 110 and CG 45) all state that continuity of care should be achieved.

Continuity of care offers the following advantages within a perinatal mental health context:

- The opportunity to develop a trusting and open relationship between the woman and her midwife increases the woman's confidence to articulate her feelings.

- The midwife is able to identify changes in the woman's behaviour or presentation across appointments.

- A woman with a pre-existing or newly developed mental illness will feel less anxious about attending appointments if her midwife is familiar.

Case Example: Nadine

Nadine, a 35-year-old woman with no family history of mental health issues, was seen by the same midwife throughout her pregnancy. She had booked for antenatal care at 11 weeks and had attended all of her appointments. Nadine had an uncomplicated vaginal birth on the birth centre and was discharged home the following day. A different midwife saw her for her first postnatal visit, but for her next visit she was visited by her named midwife who immediately identified subtle changes in her presentation. Nadine appeared anxious and was asking the same questions repeatedly. She seemed to have some difficulty in retaining information.

The midwife felt that although the changes in behaviour were subtle, the woman required further assessment the following day. On her return, the midwife noted the woman's anxiety had become more elevated. The midwife contacted the perinatal mental health team who assessed the woman at home and were able to instigate a support package that involved the woman's GP, health visitor and referral to a specialist perinatal psychologist. The early detection of signs of postnatal mental illness allowed for crucial early intervention that minimised the risk to Nadine and her baby.

Maternity services need to be organised in such a way that they promote continuity of care (National Childbirth Trust, 2015). If services are structured around the woman to promote continuity, it will optimise the midwife's ability to recognise and respond to a woman's mental health needs.

One challenge that compromises continuity is poor staffing levels. Midwives frequently cover clinics that are not 'their own' in order for women to be seen. Community teams that are not fully staffed struggle to fully implement the caseload model (where a named midwife provides continued care throughout pregnancy and birth) that they strive for and, as a consequence, continuity of care is not always achieved.

'40% of women stated that they saw different midwives at their appointments.' (RCM, 2013a)

Women have identified poor continuity of care as a barrier to them feeling able to discuss their emotional well-being (Boots Family Trust *et al*, 2013). Of course, it is also important to recognise that continuity of care must go hand in hand with sensitive and supportive care from a confident and competent midwife.

Poor continuity of care is an organisational issue that presents a challenge to midwives. Midwives must continue to strive to achieve continuity of care wherever possible, in order to facilitate the establishment of a trusting relationship within which mental health issues can be identified, discussed and responded to.

Challenge 3: Time

Another organisational challenge for midwives is the ever increasing pressure on their clinical time. The increasing birth rate, increased complexity of women's physical and social needs, combined with suboptimal staffing levels all impact on the midwife's time. Often clinic appointments are reduced to the bare minimum time slots in order to maximise the number of women seen. This will inevitably impact on the quality of care given. Women have identified that staff who appear to be busy will act as a barrier to them talking openly about their feelings during appointments (Boots Family Trust *et al*, 2013):

'After all, sometimes all that pregnant women want is a listening ear and a mouth that responds.'
(Rogers, 2014)

Women need the opportunity to discuss their emotions without the feeling that the midwife is watching the clock. When clinical time is short, it seems that mental health needs are not prioritised. Midwives have a lot to do within an antenatal appointment:

- check blood pressure

- urinalysis

- monitor foetal growth

- auscultating (non-electronic assessment through listening) the foetal heart.

There are also blood tests to take or blood test results to discuss and a long checklist of other issues that need to be discussed, including birth plans:

- infant feeding

- signs of labour

- vitamin K prophylaxis

- exercise

- signing Maternity Benefit, Maternal Exemption, Healthy Start and Sure Start forms.

If the woman has additional health needs, these will often be prioritised owing to time constraints. Postnatal care can be equally pressurised if the midwife has several visits to complete before running a clinic or antenatal class in the afternoon.

The Royal College of Midwives (RCM) and NSPCC have both recognised the need for longer appointment times (Hogg, 2013; RCM, 2014). The challenge of reduced clinical time during appointments is something that may not be within an individual midwife's power to change. However, midwives can be mindful of the need to incorporate discussions about mental health in their interactions with women during pregnancy and following the birth, and to ensure that these are clearly documented. It is also important that midwives try not to communicate their anxieties about time constraints to women.

It is useful to acknowledge the impact that working in a pressurised environment can have. The midwife should take the opportunity to reflect on their own practice and identify areas where they feel that they have been unable to identify or address a woman's emotional needs owing to their own workload.

Challenge 4: Positive resistance

There is evidence to suggest that midwives display 'positive resistance' to discussing a women's mental health during appointments (MMHA *et al*, 2013; Hogg, 2013; Boots Family Trust *et al*, 2014). There appears to be an anxiety about addressing perinatal mental health and this needs to be acknowledged, deconstructed and understood.

It is possible that the time constraints discussed above impact on the midwife's willingness to open up a conversation about a woman's mental health in case the conversation raises issues that will demand more time than the midwife is able to offer. This can potentially lead to the midwife closing the channels of communication in an attempt to minimise the chance of the woman sharing her feelings. The act of sharing can also result in extra 'work' for the midwife, such as referral and liaison, which the midwife may feel adds to a workload that is already unmanageable (Lewis & Drife, 2004).

A midwife may be reluctant to discuss mental health issues if they feel unable to resolve them (MMHA *et al*, 2013):

'The services are not there to support women and why open a can of worms that you can do nothing about.'
(Community midwife, Boots Family Trust *et al*, 2013)

Midwives experience the sense of not wanting to ask questions about mental health because they don't want to hear the answer if it means raising a problem that cannot be easily solved. Indeed, a lack of clear pathways of referral can be hugely problematic for midwives as they are then unsure of what action to take if a woman does vocalise her emotional distress.

It is important that midwives are aware of the local pathways outlining how and where to refer women if they are experiencing mental health difficulties.

Challenge 5: Interfaces with mental health services

A recent review of perinatal services in the UK displayed a shocking deficiency in the availability of specialist care for women. There are huge inconsistencies in service provision across geographical areas (MMHA, 2014). This report highlighted that 73% of NHS trusts do not employ a specialist mental health midwife and 50% of trusts do not have a perinatal mental health team with a specialist psychiatrist (Hogg, 2013). This presents further challenges to midwives who have to negotiate significant gaps in service provision in order to refer women appropriately.

Another challenge presented to midwives where there is a lack of specialist perinatal mental health services is the interplay between midwifery and mental health services. Each profession has its own culture, with its own language and its own thresholds, which can cause considerable difficulties when these services interface. Community mental health teams may well have higher thresholds for concern about treatment or urgency of referral for a woman than maternity or perinatal services, which will be holding her baby in mind.

Case example: thresholds for concern

A midwife working on a busy postnatal ward noticed that a woman had a 'funny turn' and appeared to be 'spaced out' and 'didn't know where she was'. The midwife was sufficiently concerned to contact the hospital liaison psychiatry team. The liaison team declined to see the woman as she was not suicidal or expressing any features of psychosis. They suggested that the woman may have been tired and experiencing the effects of medications given in labour and advised the midwives to let her sleep. Within six hours, the woman developed postnatal psychosis and was sectioned under the Mental Health Act (2007).

This case, although extreme, will resonate with the familiar feeling of frustration for midwives when their concerns are not acknowledged or acted upon. There are certainly training issues raised in this example, as the midwife was not able to articulate her concerns in a way that would alert the liaison team to the degree of concern. In addition, the liaison team would also have assessed the situation without the benefit of specialist perinatal knowledge. This demonstrates that there can be complexities within the relationship between midwifery and psychiatry, when they should be working seamlessly together to provide safe care for women. The employment of a specialist perinatal mental health midwife and specialist perinatal psychiatric team would serve to promote joint working between midwifery and mental health services and therefore minimise the service failures in the above example (MMHA *et al*, 2013).

Challenge 6: Complex physical health needs

Along with the increasing birth rate, there is also an increase in the complexity of the physical health needs that midwives encounter in women around the time of delivery.

The most recent MBRRACE report highlights several significant health issues (MBRRACE-UK, 2014). These include:

- sepsis
- influenza
- obesity
- haemorrhage
- thromboembolic disorder
- diabetes
- pre-eclampsia
- coexisting medical disorders such as epilepsy, heart disease and cancer.

Midwives are also caring for a growing number of women over the age of 40, which presents a new set of challenges (RCM, 2013b; RCOG, 2009). Although midwives will always work in partnership with the obstetric team when caring for women with complex physical needs, the detection and management of these conditions forms the template for antenatal and postnatal care. Therefore, in terms of the management of clinical time within appointments, addressing these physical needs is prioritised. In addition, more and more clinical resources are being configured around meeting these needs. For example, the provision of specialist clinics for obesity, diabetes, vaginal birth after caesarean (VBAC) and obstetric medicine all serve to reinforce a culture where physical health needs are paramount. This is of course in conflict with the fact that perinatal mental illness remains one of the leading causes of maternal death in the UK. A significant change in culture needs to take place, whereby the physical and mental health needs of women are addressed equally within maternity services.

Challenge 7: Complex social needs

The increase in complex physical health needs is mirrored by an increase in diverse complex social needs. Midwives are very aware of the importance of identifying and addressing these needs. It is now not uncommon for midwives to provide care to women who are experiencing social issues such as:

- domestic abuse

- substance misuse

- trafficking

- asylum difficulties

- migration with no recourse to public funds

- female genital mutilation (FGM)

- social isolation

- homelessness

- poverty.

Each of these issues can have a profound impact on the woman and her baby. Midwives need to approach these women with great sensitivity to the emotional impact that is inextricably linked to their complex social needs. Midwives must also acknowledge that different social needs may impact on a woman's ability to care for her baby and especially to meet his or her emotional needs.

Midwives have a professional responsibility to assess a woman's social needs in order to identify any safeguarding issues (HM Government, 2013). It is a mandatory requirement for midwives to receive regular safeguarding supervision and specialist training in this area. However, safeguarding still provokes feelings of anxiety in many midwives who may show reluctance in addressing these issues as a result. However, if social needs are overlooked, further opportunity to identify and offer appropriate emotional support may be missed.

It is interesting that 34% of women who experienced perinatal mental health issues stated that they did not share their feelings as they were afraid that their baby would be taken into care (Boots Family Trust *et al*, 2013). This highlights a real anxiety for women about the potential negative outcomes of engaging with services and one that midwives need to be mindful of.

Another significant issue is the increase in economic migration and migration secondary to military conflict. There are a number of women who do not have English as their first language who find themselves in a healthcare system that they do not understand and in which their voices aren't always heard. This should be highlighted as a huge area of risk, as these women will not be able to articulate their feelings to healthcare professionals unless there is an adequate interpreting service. Mental health often has significant cultural stigma and this means that it is essential for midwives to utilise an interpreter that is not a member of the woman's family or community. Although huge steps have been taken to meet the needs of providing interpreters within maternity services, more can be done to ensure that mental health issues are addressed fully and in a culturally sensitive way (NICE, 2014). See Chapter 8 for more on supporting women with complex social needs.

Challenge 8: Breastfeeding

Another significant public health issue that midwives have a key role in promoting is that of breastfeeding. The benefits of breastfeeding are widely documented. NHS trusts are working towards achieving the standards of breastfeeding support set out by UNICEF's Baby Friendly Initiative (UNICEF, 2012).

Supporting women in their choices around infant feeding is an important part of a midwife's role, and discussions and information sharing about breastfeeding will begin antenatally (NICE, 2008). This can present a challenge when midwives are supporting women who are experiencing mental illness. Midwives will need to be aware of issues such as the type of medication being prescribed and the woman's support network. This is particularly relevant if tiredness has been identified as a trigger for relapse. It is really important to ensure that any discussions around breastfeeding take place collaboratively between the woman, her midwife and/or obstetrician and a specialist mental health service. Mental health services should be mindful of the woman's wish to breastfeed and should prescribe medication that is not harmful to the baby via breast milk. The current NICE guidelines state that professionals should:

'Discuss breastfeeding with all women who may need to take psychotropic medication in pregnancy or in the postnatal period. Explain to them the benefits of breastfeeding, the potential risks associated with taking psychotropic medication when breastfeeding and with stopping some medications in order to breastfeed. Discuss treatment options that would enable a woman to breastfeed if she wishes and support women who choose not to breastfeed.'
(NICE, 2014)

It is hugely commendable that NICE have incorporated guidance for professionals regarding breastfeeding. For women with a known history of mental illness, any pre-birth planning needs to involve collaboration between the woman, the midwives, the obstetricians and the mental health team. Paediatricians are also a valuable source of advice and support. Midwives do not need to make these plans without input from other professionals. The aim is to formulate an infant feeding plan that centres around the woman's informed choices.

Case example: Laura

Laura was pregnant with her fourth child. She had developed postnatal psychosis following the births of each of her previous children. In collaboration with the specialist perinatal mental health team, she was prescribed medication during pregnancy with a plan to commence additional medication following the birth. Laura had never been able to breastfeed when she was ill previously. She was very clear that she intended to breastfeed this time. A complicating factor was that tiredness had been identified as a key trigger for her relapse and that she was taking medication at night that made her drowsy. In discussion with her partner, Laura made a plan that during the day she would breastfeed and also express breast milk to store in the fridge. This enabled her partner to offer their new baby feeds of expressed breast milk overnight. The fact that Laura had formulated her own feeding plan, and that her midwife and perinatal mental health team supported this plan, enabled her to breastfeed. Not only did Laura avoid a relapse in her postnatal mental illness, but she was also delighted to be able to sustain breastfeeding for the first year of her child's life.

This example demonstrates the positive impact of facilitating informed choice when formulating plans for breastfeeding. It also highlights the importance of a woman having access to specialist advice from a perinatal mental health team who can work collaboratively with the woman and the maternity services. NICE states that the woman and the healthcare professionals working with her should have 'access to specialist expert advice on the risks and benefits of psychotropic medication during pregnancy and breastfeeding' (NICE, 2014).

It is really important for the midwife to remember that she has the support of a wider network of professionals with specialist knowledge that she can access in order to support women with mental illness in their infant feeding choices. (See more about feelings towards feeding in Chapter 6.)

Conclusion

This chapter has named some of the main challenges that midwives face when providing care to women who are experiencing mental health needs.

Some of the challenges cannot be addressed without significant cultural changes in the way that maternity services are configured and deployed. There are now strong voices among professional bodies that are advocating for this change and it seems that the government is being proactive in addressing these needs.

However, it is essential that midwives do not allow themselves to be defeated by these challenges. Midwifery is a strong and resourceful profession with a long history of 'being with' childbearing women in all sorts of adverse circumstances. Being with women whose motherhood journey is coloured by mental health difficulties is a current challenge that can be met. Midwives are capable of reflecting on the demands that are made of them in their daily practice and finding ways to provide care of the highest quality that places equal emphasis on women's physical and emotional needs.

References

Bauer A, Parsonage M, Knapp M, Iemmi V & Adelaja B (2014) *The Costs of Perinatal Mental Health Problems*. Available at: www.centreformentalhealth.org.uk/costs-of-perinatal-mh-problems [online] (accessed April 2016).

Boots Family Trust, Netmums, Institute of Health Visiting, Tommy's & the Royal College of Midwives (2013) *Perinatal Mental Health Experiences of Women and Health Professionals* [online]. Available at: www.tommys.org/file/Perinatal_Mental_Health_2013.pdf (accessed April 2016).

British Psychological Society (2014) *Mental Health Training for Midwives Pledged* [online] Available at: www.bps.org.uk/news/mental-health-training-midwives-pledged (accessed April 2016).

Department of Health (1993) *Changing Childbirth: Report of the Expert Committee on Maternity Care*. London: HMSO.

Department of Health (2013) *Boost in Specialist Mental Health Midwives to Combat Post-Natal Depression: Government Statement* [online]. Available at: www.gov.uk/government/news/boost-in-specialist-mental-health-midwives-to-combat-post-natal-depression-government-statement (accessed April 2016).

HM Government (2013) *Working Together to Safeguard Children: A guide to inter-agency working to safeguard and promote the welfare of children* [online]. Available at: https://www.gov.uk/government/uploads/system/uploads/attachment_data/file/417669/Archived-Working_together_to_safeguard_children.pdf (accessed April 2016).

Hogg S (2013) *Prevention in Mind. All babies count: Spotlight on perinatal mental health* [online]. London: NSPCC. Available at: https://www.nspcc.org.uk/services-and-resources/research-and-resources/2013/all-babies-count-spotlight-perinatal-mental-health/ (accessed April 2016).

Knight M, Tuffnell D, Kenyon S, Shakespeare J, Gray R & Kurinczuk JJ (Eds) (2015) *Saving Lives, Improving Mothers' Care – Surveillance of maternal deaths in the UK 2011-13 and lessons learned to inform maternity care from the UK and Ireland Confidential Enquiries into Maternal Deaths and Morbidity 2009-13*. MBRACE-UK. Oxford: National Perinatal Epidemiology Unit, University of Oxford.

Lewis G & Drife J (2004) *Confidential Enquiry into Maternal and Child Death: Improving care for mothers, babies and children: Why mothers die 2000–2002* [online]. London: RCOG; cited in Adams H (2012) Can health visitors succeed in delivering a maternal mental health service in the absence of fidelity to a model/pathway? http://media.dh.gov.uk/network/231/files/2012/08/MMH-pathway-article.pdf (accessed April 2016).

Maternal Mental Health Alliance, NSPCC & Royal College of Midwives (2013) *Specialist Mental Health Midwives: What they do and why they matter* [online]. Available at: www.baspcan.org.uk/files/MMHA%20SMHMs%20Report.pdf (accessed April 2016).

Maternal Mental Health Alliance (MMHA) (2014) *Call to Act* [online]. Available at: http://everyonesbusiness.org.uk/wp-content/uploads/2014/07/Call-to-ACT.pdf (accessed April 2016).

MBRRACE-UK (2014) S*aving Lives, Improving Mothers' Care: Lessons learned to inform future maternity care from the UK and Ireland Confidential Enquiries into Maternal Deaths and Morbidity 2009–2012* [online]. Available at: https://www.npeu.ox.ac.uk/downloads/files/mbrrace-uk/reports/Saving%20Lives%20Improving%20Mothers%20Care%20report%202014%20Full.pdf (accessed January 2016).

Morris S (2015) 'Chain of failings' led to death of Charlotte Bevan and her newborn baby, coroner rules. *The Guardian* **9 October**.

National Childbirth Trust (2015) *Mind the Gap: Perinatal mental health service provision* [online]. Available at: www.nct.org.uk/sites/default/files/related_documents/328-NCT-mindTheGap-shortReport-loRes.pdf (accessed April 2016).

National Institute for Health and Care Excellence (NICE) (2008, modified 2014) *Antenatal Care* [online]. Available at: https://nice.org.uk/guidance/cg62 (accessed April 2016).

National Institute for Health and Care Excellence (NICE) (2014) *Antenatal and Postnatal Mental Health: Clinical management and service guidance* [online]. NICE guideline CG192. Available at: www.nice.org.uk/guidance/cg192 (accessed April 2016).

NHS Education for Scotland (2006) *Perinatal Mental Health Curricular Framework* [online]. Available at: www.nes.scot.nhs.uk/media/10161/Perinatal%20Curricular%20FW%20Final.pdf (accessed April 2016).

NSPCC (2012) *Breakdown or Breakthrough? How to support parents affected by mental health problems in the perinatal period* [online]. Available at: www.nspcc.org.uk/breakthrough (accessed April 2016).

Nursing and Midwifery Council (2009) *Standards for Pre-registration Midwifery Education* [online]. Available at: www.nmc-uk.org/Educators/Standards-for-education/Standards-for-pre-registration-midwifery-education/ (accessed April 2016).

Nursing and Midwifery Council (2016) Information request.

Press Association (2014) *More Emphasis Needed on Mental Health of Mothers, say Midwives* [online]. Available at: www.nursingtimes.net/nursing-practice-specialisms-midwifery-and-neonatal-nursing-/more-emphasis-on-mental-health-of-mothers-needed-say-midwives/5067857.article (accessed April 2016).

Rogers J (2014) *A Womb with a View: Antenatal depression* [online]. Available at: www.feministtimes.com/a-womb-with-a-view-antenatal-depression/ (accessed April 2016).

Ross-Davie M, Elliot S, Sakar A & Green L (2006) A public health role in perinatal mental health: are midwives ready? *British Journal of Midwifery* **14** (6) 330–334.

Rowan C, McCourt C & Bick D (2010) Provision of perinatal mental health services in two English strategic health authorities: Views and perspectives of the multi-professional team. *Evidence Based Midwifery* **8** (3) 98–106.

Royal College of Midwives (2013a) *State of Maternity Services Report 2012* [online]. Available at: https://www.rcm.org.uk/sites/default/files/State%20of%20Maternity%20Services%20report%202012.PDF (accessed April 2016).

Royal College of Midwives (2013b) *Number of Older Mothers Increasing* [online]. Available at: https://www.rcm.org.uk/news-views-and-analysis/news/number-of-older-mothers-increasing (accessed April 2016).

Royal College of Midwives (2014) *Maternal Mental Health: Improving emotional wellbeing in postnatal care* [online]. Available at: https://www.rcm.org.uk/sites/default/files/Pressure%20Points%20-%20 Mental%20Health%20-%20Final_0.pdf (accessed April 2016).

Royal College of Midwives (2015) *Caring for Women with Mental Health Problems: Standards and competency framework for specialist maternal mental health midwives* [online]. Available at: https:// www.rcm.org.uk/sites/default/files/Caring%20for%20Women%20with%20Mental%20Health%20 Difficulties%2032pp%20A4_h.pdf (accessed April 2016).

Royal College of Midwives (n.d.) *i-learn and i-folio*. Available at: https://www.rcm.org.uk/i-learn-and-i-folio (accessed April 2016).

Royal College of Obstetricians and Gynaecologists (2009) *RCOG statement on Later Maternal Age* [online]. Available at: www.rcog.org.uk/en/news/rcog-statement-on-later-maternal-age (accessed April 2016).

Sandall J (2014) *The Contribution of Continuity of Midwifery Care to High Quality Maternity Care*. London: Royal College of Midwives [online]. Available at: https://www.rcm.org.uk/sites/default/files/ Continuity%20of%20Care%20A5%20Web.pdf (accessed April 2016).

Underdown A & Barlow J (2012) *Maternal Emotional Wellbeing and Infant Development: A good practice guide for midwives* [online]. London: Royal College of Midwives. Available at: https://www.rcm. org.uk/sites/default/files/Emotional%20Wellbeing_Guide_WEB.pdf (accessed April 2016).

UNICEF (2012) *Guide to the Baby Friendly Initiative Standards* [online]. Available at: http://www. unicef.org.uk/Documents/Baby_Friendly/Guidance/Baby_Friendly_guidance_2012.pdf (accessed April 2016).

Chapter 12: Challenges for health visitors

Gemma Caton

The health visiting context

In order to discuss the challenges faced by health visitors in respect of supporting women with postnatal depression, it is helpful to consider the requirements of the health visiting role. The health visitor is often required to be a professional expert, risk assessor, patient listener, mediator, chief liaison officer and agent of change for all families. The health visiting profession often has the closest and most long-standing relationships with families in the community with children under five, and is required particularly to focus services on the families most in need. In addition to this, the current demands on, and thresholds for other services, such as adult mental health services and children's services, often mean that the health visitor is the main source of support for many families.

The Healthy Child Programme (Department of Health, 2009) sets out the services that health visiting and other early years providers should be delivering to families with children from pre-birth until five years old. The programme stipulates a schedule for routine screening, contact, advice and interventions that aims to improve the health, social and educational outcomes for children. The programme reflects the extensive research evidence discussed in Chapter 6, which recognises the lifelong impact of early childhood experiences on future adult emotional and social functioning. In conjunction with this, the National Health Visiting Service Specification 2014/15 (NHS England, 2014) outlines specifically how the health visiting service will deliver the Healthy Child Programme. New guidance from NICE (2014) stipulates that health visitors and health professionals should be asking women at every contact about their mental health and well-being, both in the antenatal and postnatal period.

Parental mental health and parenting

One of the key aims of the Healthy Child Programme and the Health Visiting Service Specification is to help parents develop strong bonds with their children.

Poor parental mental health is identified as a key element that adversely affects this bonding process and the programme highlights the importance of early identification and assessment of risk in respect of this. Both documents highlight several evidence-based models of practice and intervention – such as the Solihull Approach (Douglas & Ginty, 2001) and Video Interaction Guidance (Kennedy *et al*, 2011) – for health visitors to potentially utilise when supporting families to promote a positive bonding experience between them and their baby. These will be discussed later on in the chapter.

Health visitor listening visits

When parental mental health issues are detected, and there is a particular emphasis on identification of postnatal depression because of its known adverse impact on child development, then health visitor listening visits are recommended. Listening visits consist of six to eight contacts of one hour in duration and are based on the principles of active and reflective listening (Segre *et al*, 2010). The purpose of the visits can also be understood in terms of the concept of containment (discussed in Chapter 6), whereby the mother who is overwhelmed by her own anxious, angry and frightening feelings is listened to and given a sense that those feelings have been heard and understood. This process restores in the mother the ability to think and reflect. In this way, containing the mother's feelings restores in her the ability to contain the feelings of her infant.

Health visiting has long recognised listening visits as an important part of the role, but they may represent several challenges for health visitors on the ground:

1. Listening visits are based on sound therapeutic principles of which health visitors may have limited understanding, as this is not currently a mandatory part of the health visiting training.

2. Research tells us that while postnatal depression can result in disturbances in a parent-infant attachment relationship, alleviating the depression alone does not reduce the difficulty for the child owing to the impact of depression on this co-constructed relationship. Therefore, health visitors have to be mindful of the infant's emotional experience as well as the mother's.

3. Health visiting has historically been based around a medical model of practice, where medical difficulties are identified and health visitors are required to 'advise' families of the ways to manage such difficulties; it could be argued that this does not easily sit alongside the idea of 'listening'.

4. In order to listen effectively, health visitors need to feel contained themselves and achieving this while meeting the demands of a busy and challenging caseload can be difficult.

5. Working with people who are depressed can take its toll. Perceptions of and access to good clinical supervision for health visitors is patchy across organisations.

6. Even though the Healthy Child Programme and the National Health Visiting Service Specification 2014/2015 (NHS England, 2014) include recommendations for health visitors regarding the promotion of effective models of intervention for, and the promotion of, secure attachment, access to this training varies considerably across the country. In addition, some areas have developed specialist perinatal infant mental health services with specialist health visiting and midwifery roles to deliver and support this training while some have not.

7. Supporting families whose spoken language is not English is difficult, but listening visits undertaken via an interpreter are extremely difficult.

8. Listening visits may not be seen as a priority when organisations face staff vacancies and recruitment issues.

Taking responsibility for the challenge

Despite these challenges, it can be argued that many health visitors demonstrate a good deal of passion, understanding and commitment to supporting women and families where poor mental health adversely affects parenting. Owing to the timing of their visits, health visitors are in an excellent position to identify low mood, anxiety and other mental health difficulties – not just in the postnatal period but antenatally as well – and to offer support through timely listening visits that are mindful and inclusive of the infant's emotional experience, and, where necessary, to refer and signpost women and their partners to other organisations for support (see discussion of referral pathways in Chapter 13).

Within the recommendations of the Healthy Child Programme, health visitors are given a certain level of autonomy in which to manage the needs of their clients and the needs of the service. While all of these challenges directly face the health visitor 'on the ground', it is perhaps important to think about which of these challenges belong to the health visitor and which to the organisation in which the health visitor works. Correct ownership of these challenges is important in identifying which challenges the individual may be able to manage in respect of their practice and which organisational challenges would be difficult or impossible to manage without organisational support. Challenges 1–5 represent challenges that the individual health visitor can have some influence on by thinking about the management of their own practice. Challenges 6–8, however, are clearly those that need to be addressed at an organisational level.

Individual health visiting practice

With regards to the challenges that an individual practitioner may face, it could be helpful for health visitors and midwives to consider the universally accepted and understood research and literature in respect of the importance of professional and therapeutic boundaries. However, some of the ideas about therapeutic boundaries will be relevant for health visitors and some will be less relevant. Although access to training is variable across the country, many health visitors have had, or will have access to, Solihull Approach training, and many of the important ideas about therapeutic boundaries can be understood in respect of the concept of containment.

The Solihull Approach

In respect of all the challenges, an understanding of the Solihull Approach (Douglas & Ginty, 2001; Douglas & Brennan, 2004) is essential (see http://solihullapproachparenting.com/). This approach helps us to appreciate not only the importance of an infant's early emotional experience in relation to its parents and in respect of future emotional and social functioning, but all our relationships, especially those with our clients and our relationships within our organisations.

The approach encompasses three main principles that are all interlinked: containment, reciprocity and behaviour management (see Figure 12.1). Containment is based on the concept as described by Bion (1967), who first considered the concept of containment when thinking about the mother-infant relationship. In its simplest terms, this can be described as the mother's ability to accept, think about and make sense of her infant's many emotions (she becomes a container for these emotions), in turn allowing the infant to assemble thoughts of his own. Development of the infant's mind comes from his mother's ability to help him bear and make sense of actual difficult experiences, rendering them tolerable to the infant, and leaving him with a sense that he can be understood and tolerated (contained). Thus, in the opposite of this, a mother who is unable to tolerate or think about her infant's emotions leaves the infant not only with his original frightening feelings but with the sense that there is something intolerable about him. Where the mother does not receive this containment from external support, such as the baby's father or her own mother, or where her own mother was unable to help her feel contained as an infant, it can be argued that clients often turn to professionals for this support. Containment is primarily what a health visitor listening visit is able to provide for the mother and infant. Reciprocity refers to the quality of the parent-infant relationship. According to the Solihull Approach:

'Reciprocity describes the sophisticated interaction between a baby and an adult where both are involved in the initiation, regulation and termination of the interaction. Reciprocity can also be used to describe the interaction within all relationships.'
(Douglas, 2010)

Behaviour management is described as a third element that is only thought about and facilitated when there is evidence of containment and reciprocity.

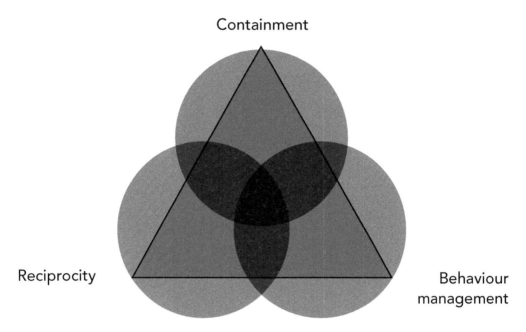

Figure 12.1: The Solihull Approach triangle. Reprinted with permission from The Heart of England NHS Foundation Trust.

Containment

Containment can be thought about in terms of offering emotional containment and understanding, but its literal sense of keeping something contained within and holding or restraining something can also be applied. In this way containment is also thought about as a barrier or boundary within which to behave, and a key function of containment in respect of the parent-infant relationship can be that of limit and boundary setting in order to keep the infant emotionally and physically safe. This also gives the infant the sense that they can be managed by the parent.

Case example: Sarah

Sarah's health visitor first began visiting her when she was six weeks postnatal with her second child Rebecca. Sarah reported feeling low and had seen her GP who had reported she had postnatal depression. The health visitor offered Sarah some listening visits so she could discuss how she was feeling and she accepted.

At each visit Sarah was keen to talk about the many difficulties she was experiencing in her relationship with her husband and mother. At the first visit her health visitor heard about the emotional neglect Sarah had suffered at the hands of her mother when she was a child. Sarah spoke about her mother's dependency on alcohol and how frequently Sarah had been left to care for herself. Sarah spoke about how this made her question her own parenting ability. The visit was longer than the hour her health visitor had planned but Sarah seemed to need the time to talk and was telling her health visitor things that were really helpful for her to know. When the visit finally came to an end Sarah said she had found it really good to talk and they arranged another visit.

The health visitor hoped that her initial time with Sarah was time well spent and that she would need to spend less time with her in the future. However, she noticed that as the weeks progressed the visits continued to last longer than an hour, often when she tried to leave Sarah would start talking about something really difficult so the health visitor felt compelled to stay and let her finish what she was saying. She felt it was important to continue to listen but this often placed strain on the rest of her day, and she noticed that she began to hear the same issues over and over again. It became harder and harder to help Sarah think about these issues or even to reflect on what had been going on. Sarah kept requesting that her health visitor return but the health visitor felt that she had become less focused and began to find it harder to listen intently; she started to feel unhelpful and overwhelmed.

Although Sarah was depressed and that was a concern, her health visitor was never concerned about the care of the children. After she had been visiting Sarah for about three months she went on leave, and then Sarah had to cancel a visit due to ill-health. When the health visitor rang her to rearrange she didn't answer so she left a message for Sarah to contact her. The health visitor's caseload got busier and she realised after a while that Sarah hadn't been in touch. She meant to follow her up but was busy with other things so relied on Sarah to contact her if she needed to. On reflection, the health visitor felt she should have ended their contact differently after all the time they had spent together, but Sarah had said she felt better and the visits had always taken up so much of her time.

In this example the health visitor has shown a commitment to Sarah and to listening to her problems, which is commendable, and it is clear that Sarah benefited from this care. However, it also appears that the visits were lengthy and had become unfocused and at times unhelpful. The ending of the visits was abrupt. It is not clear what Sarah felt about this but the health visitor reflected that this left a sense of unease about things having not ended as well as they might.

In terms of containment and the related ideas about limit and boundary setting, it may well be helpful to set a time limit on 'listening' with a client and make sure that this limit is adhered to. It is helpful to think about negotiating, where possible, a set day and time for a listening visit so that a certain level of predictability can be established. It is this predictability and consistency that can make a client feel safe enough to explore difficult feelings, and to prevent the professional from being overwhelmed.

Reciprocity

The concept of reciprocity helps us to keep in mind the important element of the parent-infant relationship, and the relationship we have in turn with the client. It has been previously shown that listening visits offer containment to adults who can feel 'uncontained'. When managing a client relationship it is very important that the adult feels listened to and understood, but health visitors face the further complexity that for them the child's best interest is paramount, and in this way the infant or child's emotional experience will also need to be thought about and understood. When listening to an adult describe their difficulties, it is helpful to name some of this emotional experience to a client but it may also be useful to 'wonder' with a parent what their infant's experience of this emotionally difficult time might be. The parent may not be able to respond immediately to these 'wonderings', but the idea of an infant with an emotional world of their own is highlighted and this is of vital importance for the infant in order that they are not 'forgotten' by the parent who is overwhelmed by their own emotional difficulties. Outside of the therapeutic frame of the listening visit there are now several resources available that can help health visitors to support parents to think about their infant's emotional world. The Solihull Approach helps parents to think about the 'dance' of reciprocity. That is, the elements that make up an enjoyable and comfortable interaction with the infant.

Behaviour management

Giving advice is an important aspect of a health visitor's role and of course many families will find this useful. In respect of managing a child's behaviour, parents often want a quick fix, and health visitors can be drawn into giving behaviour management advice when not enough is known about the parent's ability to contain the child's emotions, or the quality of the relationship between the parent and child. Under this sort of pressure to react, it may be helpful for the health visitor to reinforce the nature of the visits, and keep these separate from any sessions involving other aspects of the health visiting role. This may then free the health visitor to listen and resist the urge to give advice. If clients are given time and space to reflect and think, they can often come up with their own solutions and in this way any change is more likely to be followed through, thus reducing the likelihood of continued health visitor involvement.

A mother's own attachment history

As discussed previously in Chapter 6, parents' own attachment relationships and their experience of being parented will create a template or expectation of how all future relationships will be. A woman's earliest experience of a female authority figure is most likely to be with her own mother and, as a largely female profession, it is important for health visitors as female authority figures to consider to what extent this previous experience may help or hinder their current relationship with their client. Where early relationships have been good, it is likely that the client is already expecting the relationship with the health visitor to be positive, supportive and helpful. Where early experiences have been difficult, the client may have an altogether different expectation of the health visitor, perhaps as someone who is critical and judgemental, or preoccupied and unavailable.

In the previous case example ('Sarah') the health visitor was not clear about the time limit or the boundaries of her visit with Sarah, and she was keen to push the time that the health visitor had to offer. It is possible that even if the health visitor had set a time limit, Sarah would have found this difficult to manage. This might be as a result of her not having had boundaries set for her in her infancy or in respect of feeling a need to get as much care from the health visitor as possible, again, due to a lack of care in her infancy and a sense that care would not always be available. The health visitor worked conscientiously to support Sarah but may have inadvertently repeated patterns of behaviour from Sarah's past by not setting an appropriate boundary on her behaviour. Because a boundary was not set and reinforced, the health visitor increasingly found herself pushed for time when visiting Sarah and this eventually led to the health visitor being less proactive in the ending of the sessions. Because of this, Sarah may have had a sense of someone in a caring position ending their care abruptly and not being able to set and maintain boundaries for her, in a way that was reminiscent of her early difficult experiences.

Where early experiences have been difficult, an individual's behaviour is likely to be unconsciously motivated towards protecting themselves from future relationship difficulties based on their expectation of how relationships have gone before. In conjunction with this, they will also be drawn to continually seeking out care for themselves. Depending on previous experience this can place an individual in a conflict of wanting to get help for themselves but feeling ambivalent about engaging with help when it is offered.

Case example: Cassie

Cassie presented herself at the children's centre requesting support. She reported that she had been feeling overwhelmed and anxious much of the time. She found herself struggling to be motivated to care for her baby daughter, Chloe, who was four months old. She felt guilt about this as she felt her mother didn't care very well for her and she wanted things to be different for her daughter.

A parent–infant mental health specialist (PIMHS) picked up her case and spoke to Cassie about what support might be helpful. It was agreed that the worker would visit Cassie at home every Wednesday at 2pm for the next four weeks, so Cassie and the worker could think about Cassie's relationship with her daughter. The worker felt positive about the plan and confident that she and Cassie could work well, despite a conversation with the health visitor who had previously tried to offer Cassie more support but reported that this had not been taken up. The first session went well. The worker asked Cassie to tell her about her family tree and Cassie talked at length about her early history. The worker came away with a better understanding of Cassie's experience and felt it was important that Cassie had been able to express something of her distress and sadness at what she had previously experienced. However, Cassie was not in for the next session. When she was contacted to rearrange the session she reported that she had forgotten about it, but she was then late for the next session. At the third session, Cassie was at home but had a friend with her.

After supervision, the PIMHS was helped to understand Cassie's ambivalence towards her and rejection of her. In this way she was able to persist and eventually managed to engage Cassie so that positive steps forward were made.

In order to change a client's expectations of relationships, it is important that the professional maintains a thoughtful, reflective and consistent approach, maintaining appointments and keeping to time despite these difficulties, and despite, perhaps, the client's rejection of these attempts. While a face-to-face interaction is preferable, it may be that an arrangement has been made to contact a client by telephone in order that the practitioner 'keeps in touch' with them. This can have an important function of 'holding the client in mind', in the same way that we would wish a parent to hold their baby in mind. If this arrangement is made, it is important that the practitioner sticks to the plan even if the client does not respond, so that the client does not face a sense of rejection in the here and now, or the absence of holding in mind does not inadvertently reinforce an unconscious sense that that they have been forgotten, or are not worthy of being remembered.

Other approaches

The Newborn Behavioural Observations System (2005) helps parents and clinicians to notice and reflect together on an infant's states of emotional arousal. Close observation using the Newborn Behavioural Observations System (NBO) gives parents a wealth of specific information about their infant's individual characteristics and how they can support the infant's emotional world as he or she continues to grow and develop. Video Interaction Guidance (Kennedy *et al*, 2011), often referred to as VIG, similarly helps parents to reflect on joyful moments of interaction with their infants so they may replicate these again and again. All of these approaches are enriching and useful, and it is stipulated in the Health Visiting Specification that they should be used to enhance health visiting practice. However, individual health visitors can, and do, make a difference just by noticing with a parent an infant's preference for face-to face contact when it happens in front of them, for example, or noticing with a parent when an infant isn't enjoying some aspect of an interaction.

The pressure to 'fix it'

It can be argued that in times of anxiety and stress it is not only parents who want a 'quick fix' for a family's issues. As previously mentioned, despite a recent recruitment drive, health visitors' caseloads are still large. A family's needs can be varied and complex, and health visitors may feel the need to unconsciously defend themselves from the emotional difficulties of a client by giving them practical ways of managing those difficulties in the form of advice. As many health visitors will know, in this situation the advice is rarely taken up! The health visitor may be working with 10, 20 or even higher numbers of families with a complex level of need, while at the same time adhering to the schedule of contacts for all families within their given caseload. If listening visits are linked to the role of containment and health visitors are containing anxiety and stress for a number of families, then who contains them? This highlights the necessity for good clinical supervision. Good quality and regular clinical supervision not only restores in the practitioner the ability to think, so they can think with the client, but enables them to think with the supervisor about the relationship between themselves and the client, and what complex conscious or unconscious processes may be being played out.

Organisational challenges

This then brings us to the challenges of supporting women with postnatal depression that belong to the health visitor's organisation. Despite the increased understanding over the last 20 years of the effects of postnatal depression on child development and the importance of early attachment relationships, it can be argued that some organisations responsible for providing care for women and children have been slow to respond to this evidence. In addition, there exists a national issue of working therapeutically with clients whose first language is not English or who have no English at all. Health visitors on the ground need the containment that is provided by clear care pathways and referral routes for parents with poor mental health, and access to training and supervision if they are to be able to most effectively contain and support the attachment relationships of the clients with whom they work. It is essential that health visitors continue to highlight this to their organisations and find like-minded individuals across organisations who are equally interested in improving these services for families. The development of perinatal mental health networks that can promote this is explored in the next chapter.

Conclusion

In conclusion, health visitors face a number of challenges when supporting women with postnatal depression and where other circumstances are impacting on the development of a secure attachment relationship between them and their child. This chapter has given an overview of the complexities of the health visiting role, highlighted some of the challenges, and suggested ways in which the individual health visitor can think about and organise their practice so as to make the most positive impact with the families with whom they work. It has also highlighted where organisations that deliver health visiting and other health and social care services need to work together to support the health visitor to support families. Finally, the potential relationship the health visitor develops with a family is fairly unique to the health visiting role; if health visitors are supported, it is this relationship that has the power to strengthen and support the parent-infant relationship, assuring improved outcomes for future generations.

References

Bion W (1967) *Second Thoughts: Selected papers on psycho-analysis*. London: Maresfield Reprints.

Department of Health (2009) *Healthy Child Programme: Pregnancy and the first five years of life*. London: Department of Health.

Douglas H (2010) Supporting emotional health and wellbeing: the Solihull Approach. *Community Practitioner* **83** (8) 22–25.

Douglas H & Brennan A (2004) Containment, reciprocity and behaviour management; preliminary evaluation of a brief early intervention (the Solihull Approach) for families with infants and young children. *The International Journal of Infant Observation* **7** (10) 89–107.

Douglas H & Ginty M (2001) The Solihull Approah: changes in health visiting practice. *Community Practitioner* **74** (6) 222–224.

Kennedy H, Landor M & Todd L (Eds) (2011) *Video Interaction Guidance: a relationship-based intervention to promote attunement, empathy and wellbeing*. London: Jessica Kingsley Publishers.

National Institute for Health and Care Excellence (NICE) (2014) *Antenatal and Postnatal Mental Health: Clinical management and service guidance*. NICE clinical guideline 192. London: NICE. Available at: www.nice.org.uk/guidance/cg192 (accessed May 2016).

NHS England (2014) National Health Visiting Service Specification 2014/2015. London: NHS England.

Newborn Behavioural Observations System 2005. Boston, MA: The Brazelton Institute.

Nugent JK, Keefer CH, Minear S, Johnson L & Blanchard Y (2007) Understanding Newborn Behavior and Early Relationships: The Newborn Observations (NBO) System handbook. Baltimore: Paul H Brooks Publishing.

Segre L, Stasik S, O'Hara M & Arndt S (2010) Listening visits: an evaluation of the effectiveness and accessibility of a home-based depression treatment. *Psychotherapy Research* **20** (6) 712–721.

Solihull Community Services (2002) *Solihull Approach Resource Pack: The first five years*. Solihull: Solihull NHS Care Trust.

Chapter 13: Perinatal mental health pathways and networks

Eleanor Grant and Gemma Caton

The focus of this book has been the importance of the perinatal period for both mother and baby. This crucial time encompasses the transition to parenthood for the mother and father, and forms the foundation for ongoing development for the infant. The nature of the baby's experiences during this time will have far reaching effects. At this time, if the baby has good enough care, the foundations for emotional resilience and empathy for others will be laid. At the heart of the baby's experiences are the relationships developed with those around him or her. The development of robust, integrated services to support families in the perinatal period also depends on good relationships. As perinatal and infant mental health awareness grows, the co-ordination of burgeoning services is vital.

Most women whom midwives and health visitors support will have no significant mental health issues. Those who do are most likely to have a mild to moderate antenatal or postnatal depression and/or anxiety. In these circumstances the vast majority of women will not need a specialist service and will probably be managed in primary care by the health visitor and GP. Chapter 12 has highlighted how an understanding of basic therapeutic principles can inform and enhance this work. It has also highlighted that it is essential for professionals 'on the ground' to feel well supported in order to be most effective for the client and safe for the practitioner. However, when depression in the postnatal period is severe, when puerperal psychosis is present or when a previous neglectful, abusive or traumatic parenting experience prevents the formation of a secure attachment relationship, a specialist service will be essential. This chapter will suggest how mental health networks and care pathways can support practitioners who are 'holding' the care of infants whose mothers have mild to moderate difficulties, and how they can facilitate a smooth transition into more specialist services where appropriate.

There are many documents and policies that stipulate the need for and the essential nature of clinical networks, such as the *Antenatal and Postnatal Mental*

Health guidelines (NICE, 2014) and the *Guidance for Commissioners of Perinatal Mental Health Services* (JCPMH, 2012). These are the most recent in a long line of documents and guidance that have aimed over the last decade to inform the development of such services. However, organisational response has been slow. For example, specialist inpatient services (mother and baby units) are still few and far between. Despite the emphasis on developing services, maternal death rates from indirect causes, which include psychiatric causes, remain high with no significant change in the rate since 2003 (Knight *et al*, 2015; CMACE, 2011). Suicide is the second leading cause of maternal death after cardiovascular disease (Mental Health Taskforce, 2016).

However, there are areas of good practice. Across the country there are examples of specialist services and perinatal mental health pathways that have been developed successfully. Care pathways help improve care and outcomes for mothers and babies by offering guidance for practitioners which promotes a coherent, consistent response using enhanced multidisciplinary networks. The development of effective services requires, as a minimum, the following to be in place:

■ care pathways with clear guidance informed by best practice

■ agreed referral routes

■ relevant training for those delivering services

■ support and supervision to maintain services.

All of the above will need good working relationships and clear, strong leadership to drive forward the agenda while facilitating a supportive, compassionate culture in which new networks and services can grow.

Care pathways

As the paediatrician and psychoanalyst Donald Winnicott famously said: 'There is no such thing as an infant,' because, as a baby would not exist without a caregiver, there is always an infant and someone (Winnicott, 1960a). This remark highlights the fact that a baby does not exist in isolation. There will be many people around in various roles. The perinatal mental health sphere straddles many areas: child and adult health, mental health and social care may all be involved at some point, depending on the level of need. To find a way through the myriad services a care pathway can be useful.

A care pathway is a tool to organise healthcare decision-making for a particular group of patients. Care pathways bring together the evidence base and best practice guidelines to inform a process whereby all professionals involved in a person's care know their role and how it relates to others. The European Pathways Association (EPA) states that a care pathway is a 'complex intervention for the mutual decision making and organisation of care processes for a well-defined group of patients during a well-defined period'. The EPA website lists defining characteristics of care pathways as including:

■ *'The facilitation of the communication among team members and with patients and families.*

■ *The coordination of the care process by the coordination of roles and sequencing activities of the multidisciplinary care team, patients and their relatives.'*

(http://e-p-a.org/care-pathways/)

There is uneven provision of care pathways across the UK but several regions have implemented them in order to support development of perinatal mental health services. Scotland (SIGN, 2012), Northern Ireland (HSC, 2012) and England (DH, 2012) have all produced pathways and guidelines for maternal and infant mental health. A recent collaboration between the Association for Infant Mental Health and Warwick University resulted in a new online pathway to support professionals working with women in the perinatal period (discussed further in this chapter). Successful care pathways are the product of collaboration; they are partnerships. All the services that form part of the pathway should be represented in the development group. Ideally, the process of working together to agree pathways will result in making links between services and the development of a shared culture. Shared ownership heightens commitment to the implementation of the new ways of working. Pathways that give clear guidelines to the various professionals involved in the care process are easier to follow and more likely to be adhered to.

It is important to remember that the infant is at the heart of all this planning. The infant, who will in time become an adult and maybe a parent, is at the centre of the relationships with those around him or her. In order to optimise care for infants, the context or circumstances of the baby's life need to be considered. There is a sort of nested arrangement whereby, ideally, the baby is supported by the mother, the mother by the father and family, the family by the wider community including professionals. The professionals, in their turn, will need support in order to do their job to the best of their ability. Such support and supervision wraps around the system offering, hopefully, containment for all involved. This system can be represented by the diagram in Figure 13.1.

This simplified graphic brings to mind Urie Bronfenbrenner's ecological model of human development (1994), which considers the broader context in which an individual develops. He argues that it is not only the various systems and subsystems that affect how an individual develops but, crucially, the interaction or linkages between the various layers that are important. Bronfenbrenner's ideas were influential in the development of interventions in the US, such as Head Start, which he co-founded, and the Nurse Family Partnership. These ideas also underpinned UK initiatives, for example, the Family Nurse Partnership (FNP) and the original Sure Start (later Children's Centres) concept.

Care pathways aim to enhance communication between professionals, encourage collaboration and promote shared vision. They can provide the linkages and relationships between the various services available to the perinatal population.

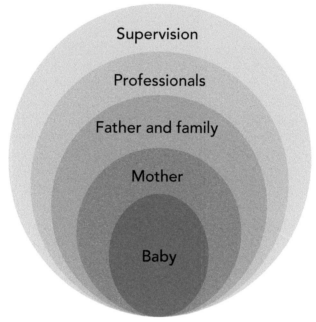

Figure 13.1: Potential sources of support around the infant

The development of care pathways continues across the country. The Association for Infant Mental Health in collaboration with Warwick University has launched an online Infant Mental Health Pathway, which aims to promote emotional well-being from the start, prevent difficulties if possible, and facilitate early responses and treatment when necessary (see: https://www2.warwick.ac.uk/fac/med/about/centres/wifwu/research/mhpathway). The stated aim is to give 'every child the best start in life by promoting the wellbeing of parents and their babies across the perinatal period'.

The Joint Commissioning Panel for Mental Health (JCPMH) *Guidance for Commissioners of Perinatal Mental Services* recommends that in every region there is an integrated care pathway to cover 'all levels of service provision and severities of disorder', not just for those requiring admission to a mother and baby unit (JCPMH, 2012).

Referral routes

The availability of care pathways enables coherent packages of care to be offered and referral routes facilitated. Collaboration is key: good relationships make for good referrals. The routes into more specialist services will need to be agreed during the pathway development in order to smooth transition from one service to another and reduce the likelihood of service users falling through gaps in service (see Khan, 2015). Some care pathways, including in Great Yarmouth and Northern Ireland, have included template letters to facilitate referral between agencies. The delivery of the Healthy Child Programme (HCP) (DH, 2009) may involve liaising and referring to specialist mental health services and, if available, specialist perinatal mental health services. The Improving Access to Psychological Therapies (IAPT) services (see www.iapt.nhs.uk) accept self-referrals, but a referral might also be made by the health visitor when a mother is not able to make contact herself.

Training

Perinatal emotional issues can easily be either dismissed as trivial (and confused with normal, fleeting experiences such as the 'baby blues') or feared as a 'can of worms', which might overwhelm both the mother and the worker. The confidence to help and the awareness of one's own limits and when referral would be advisable can be developed through good training. The national training body, Health Education England (HEE), is committed to developing training in perinatal mental health for midwives and health visitors as part of the priorities for promoting and sustaining good mental health (DH, 2014). The Royal College of General Practitioners (RCGP) has also prioritised a plan to improve GP management of perinatal mental health (Khan, 2015). These initiatives aim to improve the detection of perinatal mental health issues and enhance confidence in practitioners in responding. The RCGP report noted that women felt most positive about the care they received when they felt it was personalised and integrated, and when they experienced it as 'wrapping around their needs' (echoes of Bronfenbrenner's nested structures).

A problem highlighted by the RCGP report is the long waiting time experienced in some areas for psychological therapies. Despite the NICE guidance that perinatal women should be prioritised, the provision of psychological therapies is patchy across the UK. For a perinatal mental health care pathway to work well, and for midwives and health visitors to have confidence in it, specialist mental health services must be available for them to refer into.

Good training can raise awareness, influence the predominant culture and help overcome barriers and shift attitudes. It can also heighten awareness of treatment options available – for example, psychological therapies – and referral routes. The Institute of Health Visiting and Health Education England (HEE) are developing programmes and training to enhance skills in the workforce. HEE now offers an e-learning package on perinatal mental health (see www.e-lfh.org.uk/programmes/perinatal-mental-health).

Supervision

If good training is necessary in order to set up good services, then good supervision is necessary for the maintenance of them. Supervision can perform a 'holding' function for the professional, mirroring the holding function that the professional offers the family. Donald Winnicott (1960b) wrote about the concept of 'holding', which is essential to the infant's emotional development. When babies are 'held' in this way they can be confident that their needs will be met. In time this leads to self-confidence and emotional robustness. Like Bion's 'containment' (see Chapter 6) it makes intuitive sense. Working with families around the time of childbirth can stir up potent, primitive feelings, and a 'holding environment' can offer a space where they can be experienced, processed and thought about.

Helping parents think about what it is like to be a baby and what their baby might be experiencing ('mentalising', see Chapter 6) is part of promoting parents' reflective capacity. To do this successfully, health professionals need to be supported to reflect on their own practice. Reflective or restorative supervision has been shown to reduce burnout and stress in health visitors and increase job satisfaction and pleasure (Wallbank & Hatton, 2011). Ann Simpson (2005) talks about the role health visitors can have in responding to the mental health needs of families (most mental health needs of children will be managed in primary care) and how specialist training and supervision has a place in supporting them to work in challenging circumstances. A model of supervision that considers the impact of the child and family on the worker, and the worker on the family, allows the emotional aspects of both 'airtime'. As Ann Simpson states, professionals working with stressed families need to be in touch with what is being stirred in them. Consistent (and she emphasises consistent) supervision is important to allow exploration of the emotional content in the family – and in the professional. Regular, consistent, reflective supervision offers a safe place to explore such issues in a way that non-scheduled, reactive supervision cannot.

Supervision can also support health visitors and other health professionals not to rush in and act when perhaps what is required is an engaged, reflective stance ('don't just do something, stand there'). It can be hard to do this in a job so tied up with action, advice-giving and doing, but long ago the wisdom and importance of sitting with and bearing witness was quietly highlighted. In the time-honoured classic *A Fortunate Man*, about the life of a rural GP, John Berger comments: 'He does more than treat them when they are ill; he is the objective witness of their lives' (Berger & Mohr, 1967). Iona Heath, in her essay *The Art of Doing Nothing* (Heath, 2012) also discusses this from a GP's point of view. She points out that sometimes it seems we have no time to stop and think because we are too busy 'doing', whereas if we were to just be present and open to the other person, we might do more good. A reflective stance is equally important for other healthcare professionals and can be a significant part of what is offered to the family. Doing what can feel like 'nothing' but is actually being present and attentive can convey a sense that emotions can be communicated and thought about. A thoughtful, reflective and compassionate stance can offer containment both for families and for professionals.

Many healthcare professionals will be familiar with several different sorts of supervision. Managerial, administrative, practice teacher and safeguarding supervision are available to many workers. Increasingly, the role of supportive and restorative supervision in developing and maintaining a healthy workforce is acknowledged. The focus of restorative supervision is on the emotional impact of work on professionals. Acknowledging the impact of the emotional content of the work can help reduce avoidance of difficult issues by allowing them to be thought about.

The Institute of Health Visiting is leading a drive towards a 'fresh focus', with an emphasis on professionals developing compassionate resilience and enhanced self-care (DH & HEE, 2015). Angela Underdown, from the Warwick Infant and Family Wellbeing Unit, says in her paper on supporting parents to adopt a reflective stance: 'It is difficult for professionals to help others become more reflective without being supported to reflect on their own practice' (Underdown, 2013). Looking after oneself becomes a prerequisite of good practice, like putting the oxygen mask on oneself first before attending to the children, as we are regularly advised on airline flights. The process of supervision with emphasis on containment and reciprocity will be familiar to those who have attended Solihull Approach training (Douglas & Ginty, 2001), which many health visitors and midwives will have done. It is hoped that the emphasis and importance placed on restorative supervision will allow health visitors to notice and think about less sensitive interactions between parent and child. The aim is to help practitioners become more reflective about their own practice and less reactive with clients.

The case for reflective, restorative supervision is compelling. To offer containment to families means attending to one's own well-being and emotional resourcefulness. Compassionate, respectful care for others begins with compassionate self-care. As the culture changes and staff become more used to adopting a reflective approach themselves, it will become easier to bring these skills to bear in their work with women and their families.

Case example: Maureen

Maureen had always wanted to be a nurse. She trained straight from school and later also trained as a midwife. By the time she went on to train as a health visitor she had had three children of her own. She enjoyed her job and found it rewarding. In mid-life she found herself very busy with a full-time job, raising children and increasingly elderly parents but caring came naturally to her; it was what she did. The business of her life and the competing demands of home, family, parents and work left little time to reflect and think. Maureen liked it like that; she enjoyed feeling busy and useful and packed a lot into her day. However, she began to feel that she couldn't keep up and worked harder and harder to get through all her jobs. She began to feel exhausted and burnt-out. The job she had loved became a source of ongoing stress. There were opportunities to talk to her manager but Maureen felt that she should keep quiet and carry on.

When the opportunity arose to attend restorative supervision sessions, Maureen wasn't sure that she needed to go. In fact, it seemed like just another thing that had to be fitted into her already full schedule. However, she went along to see what it was all about. Although it felt quite odd to sit around when there was so much to be done, Maureen continued to attend. Over time she began to feel that the sessions offered a space to think about issues that were bothering her at work and which might not otherwise have been addressed. The opportunity for reflection, although it felt strange at first, helped Maureen think about her work in new ways, and she felt calmer and less stressed by her work.

Leadership and service champions

In order to drive forward and inspire change, strong leadership is necessary. Good leaders can bring teams with them and enthuse the workforce in new ways of working. The Institute of Health Visiting (iHV), the Royal College of Midwives (RCM) and the Royal College of General Practitioners (RCGP) are meeting this challenge. All these institutions have focused in recent years on developing awareness and skills in the perinatal mental health arena.

The iHV, established in 2012, has developed the role of perinatal mental health and infant mental health champions who receive special training in perinatal mental health issues and are charged with cascading the training to colleagues. The RCGP has identified a clinical champion to work with HEE to support specific perinatal mental health training for GPs. The IAPT guidance includes a specific perinatal positive practice guide (DH, 2013). All these initiatives help enhance a collaborative culture and foster good relationships.

The iHV infant mental health champions have been tasked with disseminating training regarding the promotion of secure attachment relationships. The training provides a wealth of information and material to help health visitors understand attachment relationships, and notice and promote sensitive, responsive parenting when they see it. The RCM has produced a good practice guide for midwives on maternal emotional well-being and infant development (Underdown & Barlow, 2012), which offers theoretical background and practical tips about supporting healthy parent-infant relationships.

These recent initiatives and support for restorative supervision for health visitors underline the importance of healthy working relationships in order to help support healthy family relationships. In addition, they carry the enthusiasm and passion for infant mental health work and inspire a new cohort of workers.

An example of the development of a parent-infant service: Great Yarmouth Parent Infant Mental Health Support (PIMHS) service

In the early years of the new millennium a truly innovative parent-infant service began to take shape in Great Yarmouth, Norfolk. This development was the result of real collaboration, visionary leadership and inspired management. The ensuing partnership involved the local Sure Start (later children's centre), the health visiting service and the Great Yarmouth primary care psychological service. The resulting developments, which form the foundation of the service to this day, are described here.

In 2001 the government Sure Start initiative brought funding to develop services for children and families living in areas of greatest deprivation. The original aims of the Sure Start programme were to enhance employment opportunities, improve families' physical health, and promote social, emotional and cognitive development in children. Part of this aim was to reduce the impact of postnatal depression because of its known effect on social and emotional development.

History of the service

As an area of high deprivation, Great Yarmouth became a 'trail blazer' with Sure Start in 2001. True to the original ethos of the Sure Start project, relationships were developed with local health and education providers and the community. In an early example of co-production of services, local parents were involved in determining which services and types of support should be developed for the families and professionals in this area. One of the community parents' main concerns was the high rate of depression in local mothers. Health visitors in the area had also highlighted that postnatal depression was very prevalent among the women that they were visiting, and there was little support available to meet this need. A local health needs assessment was undertaken and it was found that while the national rates of postnatal depression were thought to be about 10–15% (O'Hara & Swain, 1996), the local level of postnatal depression was found to be more like 40-50%. At this time health visitors were not routinely asking about or measuring women's mood, antenatally or postnatally; instead, the subject was introduced only if the health visitor thought this was an issue.

At the same time, separately from Sure Start, monies were made available from another fund to employ a clinical psychologist from adult mental health services to develop support for women with postnatal depression in the Great Yarmouth area. The resulting relationship between adult mental health services, health visiting and the Sure Start centre brought about a way of thinking about how to support women with postnatal depression. It was in this way that the Priory Children's Centre Parent Infant Mental Health Service (PIMHS) began.

The service had three major achievements in its first year:

■ It devised and delivered a training programme for all health visitors to identify and respond to women with postnatal depression.

■ It hosted a conference, 'Making the Links – Shaping the Future: Postnatal depression and infant mental health', in Great Yarmouth.

■ It developed an integrated care pathway for maternal depression.

The conference brought to Great Yarmouth internationally renowned speakers, to help stimulate interest and raise awareness of the impact of postnatal depression on infant mental health. This interest was harnessed by involving key stakeholders in a potential care pathway.

Care pathway development

The care pathway originally developed in 2002 has been revised over the years; the most recent version is shown in Figure 13.2 on p192. As the service continues to evolve, further changes and developments to services have taken place since this version was issued and another iteration will be released in due course.

In order for the pathway to be effective, all agencies involved in its delivery had to be involved in its development and agree to its implementation. The implementation of the pathway brought considerable change to health visiting practice, with greater responsibility on health visitors for screening for depression and anxiety. The training offered to health visitors helped build their understanding of mental health difficulties and their confidence in talking to women about these issues. It also offered an introduction to attachment theory and its relevance to working with families. The care pathway and its supporting documentation clearly laid out the health visitors' responsibilities while the training clarified boundaries, limits and when to refer on.

Health visitors were trained and encouraged to support women with mild to moderate depression with listening visits. The pathway made clear the referral routes to the GP or adult mental health services where there were concerns about self-harm, suicide or puerperal psychosis. Relationships were built with local GPs, who were invited to the conference and involved in developing the pathway. Further documentation – for example, template letters – was produced so that health visitors could easily liaise with GPs about a client's score on the Edinburgh Postnatal Depression Scale (EPDS), and GPs were primed to expect such documentation and respond to an increased number of women identified as needing to discuss their mental health worries with a family doctor.

The conference and the training were essential in raising interest and awareness of the effects of postnatal depression on an infant's developing emotional world. It highlighted the PIMHS service's aim to support attachment relationships between parents and infants. The conference and the subsequent pathway were crucial in defining the service as support for attachment relationships rather than as mental health assessment, diagnosis and/or treatment. This was reflected in a change of name at the end of the first year of the project, from the (rather cumbersome) Great Yarmouth Multi-Agency Postnatal Depression Project to the Great Yarmouth Parent Infant Mental Health Support (PIMHS) service.

Examples of interventions offered by the service can be seen in Figure 13.2. In addition to the universal provision offered by midwives, health visitors and children's centre staff, are more targeted interventions such as 'Talking Tummies' (antenatal) and 'Talking Mummies' (postnatal) groups for women identified as low in mood. More complex needs and concerns about the attachment relationship are addressed with other interventions available at the children's centre. These services now include Video Interaction Guidance (VIG), music therapy, input from the specialist Infant Mental Health health visitor, clinical psychology sessions at the children's centre or referral into specialist mental health services.

Integrated Care Pathway – Parent Infant Mental Health

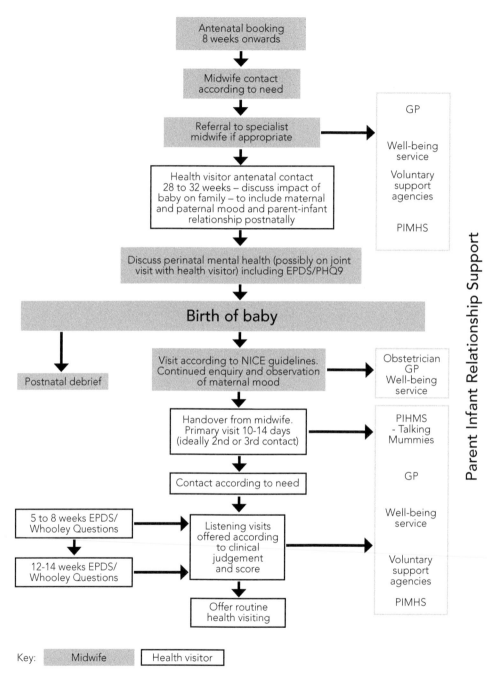

Figure 13.2. Great Yarmouth PIMHS Integrated Care Pathway 2012

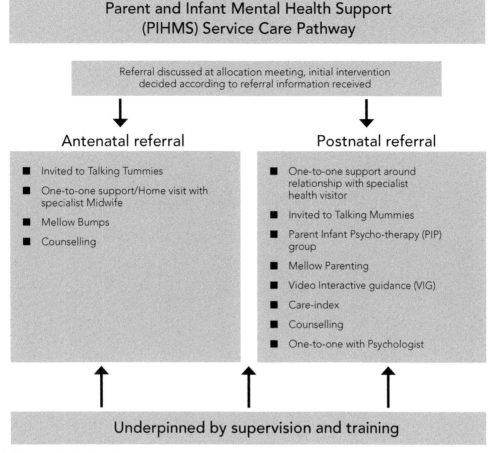

Figure 13.2 Contd.

The Great Yarmouth PIMHS service started initially with funding partly from Sure Start and partly from NHS funding for clinical psychology input. The involvement of a clinical psychologist with an adult mental health background meant that the team had both adult and child service perspectives. This psychology input enhanced a psychological understanding of parent-infant relationships, and services grew and developed according to this understanding. Over time the services in the Great Yarmouth and Waveney area have continued to evolve and continue to be innovative. The staff now includes a child and an adult psychiatrist, mental health workers and social workers. These additional disciplines bring another important dimension when thinking about and working with families, particularly those with the most complex needs. As such, the Great Yarmouth PIMHS service now offers much of the care expected in regards to maternal mental health, as recommended in the *Commissioning Mental Wellbeing for All: A toolkit for commissioners* (Newbigging & Heginbotham, 2010).

Clinical supervision in Great Yarmouth PIMHS

As highlighted by Figure 13.2, this care pathway is underpinned by training and reflective clinical supervision delivered by a psychologist. Clinical psychology time within the Great Yarmouth PIMHS service is limited, but owing to the nature and complexity and level of risk associated with the work, this time spent in supervision is essential. The collaborative relationships that underpin the care pathway and the emotional containment of supervision together offer a matrix to support the frontline staff in the team. When the workers are well supported they can in turn offer this level of emotional containment to the parent(s) and their infant. In this way, through good training and ongoing reflective supervision, PIMHS workers can 'hear the mother's cries', in order to help her hear her baby's distress (see Fraiberg, 1980 (p172) and Chapter 6, this volume).

Case example: Manuela

Manuela grew up in Portugal and had moved round the country a lot as a child. She never really felt settled anywhere. Every time she made friends it seemed that she and her family had to move on.

She had experienced some episodes of depression in her teens but by her early 20s she had a job she liked and a loving partner. However, she lost her job when the company closed and she moved to England with her partner looking for work. When she became pregnant, although it was a surprise, she was pleased and determined to give her baby a settled life and all the things she felt she had missed out on as a child. As the pregnancy progressed, she began to feel lower in mood, which made her feel guilty, as though she did not want the baby. Her partner was worried but felt helpless to change the situation; their relationship suffered.

She saw her midwife at the local children's centre and developed a good rapport with her despite the language difficulties. Her midwife noticed that her mood was slipping and invited her to the antenatal group for Portuguese mothers, which included an interpreter. The health visitor met Manuela before the birth and worked with the midwife to support her throughout the pregnancy. The local maternal mental health care pathway meant that a referral to mental health services would be facilitated if the need arose.

When the baby was born Manuela's health visitor kept a close eye on her. As they had already established a relationship it was easier for Manuela to feel she could rely on and trust her. As the professionals feared might happen, Manuela became more depressed following the birth of her baby girl. More worryingly, she had problems bonding with baby Eva. She came to the postnatal mums' group, which she found supportive, but her connection with Eva appeared fragile. Manuela appeared cut-off from her baby and the baby began to seem depressed too. The health visitor felt frustrated and found herself feeling angry with Manuela, which worried her. She discussed these feelings in supervision and was able to think about how these feelings had unsettled her. Both Manuela and her health visitor felt that they were in foreign territory.

The children's centre was able to offer Manuela parent-infant sessions with the psychologist, which aimed to support and scaffold the attachment relationship. This, along with infant massage sessions, helped Manuela begin to recognise her baby's need for her without feeling overwhelmed. Her partner was invited to the fathers' group, which increased his involvement. Manuela was able to talk about the sense of loss she had at being in a foreign country without her own mother to help her. She had felt angry and abandoned and unable to cope with the demands of a small baby. Her anger at her partner for bringing her here was also acknowledged. The health visitor understood that some of the anger she had felt had 'belonged' to Manuela. The services available at the children's centre enabled Manuela to feel looked after enough for her to find space in her mind for her infant. The team supporting her felt supported themselves through supervision and through local networks, which meant that more specialist intervention from the perinatal mental health team was available should the need arise.

Manuela's mood began to lift and baby Eva appeared more confident in her connection with her mother. Manuela later started English classes at the children's centre and signed up for childcare sessions to allow her to look for work.

Conclusion

What matters is relationships: relationships in the past can affect relationships in the present and future. The emotional health of the baby is inextricably linked with that of the mother. Attachment matters; professional relationships matter too.

Perinatal mental health is an important public health issue that concerns parent and baby, adult and child, family and community. It straddles many areas of healthcare and mothers and babies can risk falling through the gaps between services. However, services are becoming increasingly relationship-focused and the gaps are therefore being narrowed. The perinatal period is also a time when many women are in frequent contact with health services. By remembering to think about the mother's and the baby's experience, and to ask about it, well-supported staff can make sensitive enquiries about the emotional well-being of mother and baby, and can help to interrupt the cycle of disadvantage that some families seem caught in. The emotional needs of the baby, who will in time become an adult and maybe a parent, can be supported.

Support for the parent is support for the infant. Remembering Bronfenbrenner's (1994) ecological systems theory, the child and family have to be considered with reference to their environment. The cultural sensitivities of the complex context of an individual infant's life are increasingly acknowledged and services strive to become culturally relevant to the populations they serve. The current interest in perinatal and infant mental health brings a burgeoning of services dedicated to supporting the emotional well-being of new parents and their infants, and in doing so contributes to the flourishing of a new generation. As in pregnancy, despite sometimes difficult circumstances, this is a time of hope.

References

Berger J & Mohr J (1967) *A Fortunate Man*. Harmondsworth: Allen Lane, The Penguin Press.

Bronfenbrenner U (1994) Ecological models of human development. In: *International Encyclopedia of Education* (2nd edition) Vol 3. Oxford: Elsevier. Reprinted in: Gauvain M & Cole M (Eds) (1996) *Readings on the Development of Children* (2nd edition). New York: Scientific American.

Centre for Maternal and Child Enquiries (CMACE) (2011) Saving mothers' lives: reviewing maternal deaths to make motherhood safer. *British Journal of Obstetrics and Gynaecology* **118** (Supplement 1) 1–203.

Department of Health (2009) *Healthy Child Programme: Pregnancy and the first five years of life* [online]. Available at: https://www.gov.uk/government/uploads/system/uploads/attachment_data/file/167998/Health_Child_Programme.pdf (accessed April 2016).

Department of Health (2012) *Maternal Mental Health Pathway* [online]. Available at: https://www.gov.uk/government/uploads/system/uploads/attachment_data/file/212906/Maternal-mental-health-pathway-090812.pdf (accessed April 2016).

Department of Health (2013) *IAPT: Perinatal Positive Practice Guide* [online]. Available at: www.iapt.nhs.uk/silo/files/perinatal-positive-practice-guide-2013.pdf (accessed April 2016).

Department of Health (2014) *Closing the Gap: Priorities for essential change in mental health* [online]. Available at: https://www.gov.uk/government/publications/mental-health-priorities-for-change (accessed April 2016).

Department of Health & Health Education England (2015) *A National Preceptorship Framework for Health Visiting: The first two years* [online]. Available at: http://ihv.org.uk/wp-content/uploads/2015/09/iHV_preceptorshippack_V16-WEB.pdf pdf (accessed April 2016).

Douglas H & Ginty M (2001) The Solihull Approach: changes in health visiting practice. *Community Practitioner* **74** (6) 222–224.

Fraiberg S (Ed) (1980) *Clinical Studies in Infant Mental Health: The first year of life*. London: Tavistock

Heath I (2012) The art of doing nothing. *Huisarts en Wetenschap (General Practitioner and Science)* **55** (12) 580–583.

HSC (2012) *Integrated Perinatal Mental Health Care Pathway* [online]. Available at: www.publichealth.hscni.net/publications/perinatal-mental-health-care-pathway (accessed April 2016).

Joint Commissioning Panel for Mental Health (2012) *Guidance for Commissioners of Perinatal Mental Health Services* [online]. Available at: www.jcpmh.info/wp-content/uploads/jcpmh-perinatal-guide.pdf (accessed April 2016).

Khan L (2015) *Falling through the Gaps: Perinatal mental health and general practice* [online]. London: Centre for Mental Health. Available at: www.rcgp.org.uk/clinical-and-research/clinical-resources/~/media/Files/CIRC/Perinatal-Mental-Health/RCGP-Report%20-Falling-through-the-gaps-PMH-and-general-practice-March-2015.ashx (accessed April 2016).

Knight M, Tuffnell D, Kenyon S, Shakespeare J, Gray R & Kurinczuk JJ (Eds) (2015) on behalf of MBRRACE-UK. *Saving Lives, Improving Mothers' Care – Surveillance of maternal deaths in the UK 2011-13 and lessons learned to inform maternity care from the UK and Ireland Confidential Enquiries into Maternal Deaths and Morbidity 2009-13*. Oxford: National Perinatal Epidemiology Unit, University of Oxford.

Mental Health Taskforce (2016) *The Five Year Forward View for Mental Health: A report from the independent Mental Health Taskforce to the NHS in England* [online]. Available at: https://www.england.nhs.uk/wp-content/uploads/2016/02/Mental-Health-Taskforce-FYFV-final.pdf (accessed April 2016).

National Institute for Health and Care Excellence (NICE) (2014) *Antenatal and Postnatal Mental Health: Clinical management and service guidance* [online]. NICE clinical guideline 192. London: NICE. Available at: www.nice.org.uk/guidance/cg192 (accessed April 2016).

Newbigging K & Heginbotham C (2010) *Commissioning Mental Wellbeing for All: A toolkit for commissioners*. Preston: University of Central Lancashire. International School for Communities, Rights and Inclusion. Available at: http://www.mas.org.uk/uploads/100flowers/commissioning-wellbeing-for-all.pdf (accessed April 2016).

O'Hara M & Swain AM (1996) Rates and risk of postpartum depression: a meta-analysis. *International Review of Psychiatry* **8** 37–54.

Scottish Intercollegiate Guidelines Network (SIGN) (2012) *Management of Perinatal Mood Disorders: A national guideline* [online]. Available at: www.sign.ac.uk/guidelines/fulltext/127 (accessed April 2016).

Simpson A (2005) Making meaning out of the mess: Developing the mental health role of health visitors. In: J Launer, S Blake and D Daws (Eds) *Reflecting on Reality: Psychotherapists at work in primary care*. (pp132–144). London: Karnac.

Underdown A (2013) Parent–infant relationships: Supporting parents to adopt a reflective stance. *Journal of Health Visiting* **1** (2) 76–79.

Underdown A & Barlow J (2012) *Maternal Emotional Wellbeing and Infant Development: A good practice guide for midwives*. London: Royal College of Midwives.

Wallbank S & Hatton S (2011) Reducing burnout and stress: the effectiveness of clinical supervision. *Community Practitioner* **84** (7) 31–5.

Winnicott DW (1960a) The theory of the parent–infant relationship. *International Journal of Psycho-Analysis* **41** 585–595.

Winnicott DW (1960b) The relationship of a mother to her baby at the beginning. In: DW Winnicott (1965) *The Family and Individual Development*. (pp15–21) London: Tavistock.

Websites

1001 Critical Days: www.1001criticaldays.co.uk/the_manifesto.php
The 1001 Critical Days manifesto is a vision for the provision of services in the UK for the early years period, which puts forward the moral, scientific and economic case for the importance of the conception to age 2 period.

Department of Health Information Service for Parents: https://www.nhs.uk/
InformationServiceForParents/pages/faq.aspx
This service offers regular emails and/or text messages tailored to your stage of pregnancy or child's age. They cover a range of topics, including your baby's development, preparing for labour, coping with sleepless nights, looking after your own health, choosing childcare, making sure you get the benefits you're entitled to, and who's there to support you.

Health Education England (HEE) e-learning for healthcare Perinatal Mental Health: http://
www.e-lfh.org.uk/programmes/perinatal-mental-health-for-health-visitors/
The e-learning sessions are intended for use by nurses and health visitors. The three e-learning modules developed by the Institute of Health Visiting, funded by the Department of Health, look at: 1) Perinatal depression and other mental health disorders. 2) How to recognise perinatal anxiety and depression. 3) Interventions for perinatal anxiety, depression and related disorders.

Integrated Perinatal Mental Health Care Pathway Northern Ireland: http://www.publichealth.
hscni.net/publications/perinatal-mental-health-care-pathway
This regional care pathway provides guidance for all health and social care professionals in Northern Ireland who come into contact with pregnant women.

Maternal Mental Health Pathway: https://www.gov.uk/government/publications/maternal-mental-
health-pathway
Guidance on issues associated with maternal mental health and well-being, from pregnancy through the early months after the birth.

**Royal College of General Practitioners (RCGP) Clinical Priority Programme: Perinatal
Mental Health:** http://www.rcgp.org.uk/clinical-and-research/~/link.aspx?_id=DA355CAD524842FFA
B522EBE6932B5F8&_z=z
The RCGP has identified perinatal mental health as a clinical priority. It aims to develop and implement a strategy for primary care and work with partners in promoting models of best practice and pathways of care and will develop learning and educational resources.

Safer Care Pathways in Mental Health: http://mentalhealthpartnerships.com/project/safer-care-
pathways-in-mental-health-project/
The project aims to support clinical teams with care pathway improvement and clinical practice improvement in mental health care, making these pathways safer and more reliable for service users and their families.

Warwick Infant and Family Wellbeing Unit: http://www2.warwick.ac.uk/fac/med/about/centres/
wifwu/
Warwick Infant and Family Wellbeing Unit (WIFWU) brings together expertise with the goal of providing research, training and innovation in effective evidence-based ways of supporting parenting during pregnancy and the first two years of life, in order to promote the social, emotional and psychological development of infants.

Warwickshire Infant Mental Health Pathway: http://www2.warwick.ac.uk/fac/med/about/centres/
wifwu/research/mhpathway
The pathway is divided into three time periods: pre-conception, antenatal and postnatal. Each section starts with an overview of the aims and objectives for each of the time periods and then presents examples of evidence-based or promising initiatives that should be provided and references to the relevant evidence.

BV - #0051 - 060521 - C2 - 246/185/13 - PB - 9781910366295 - Gloss Lamination